Finding Home

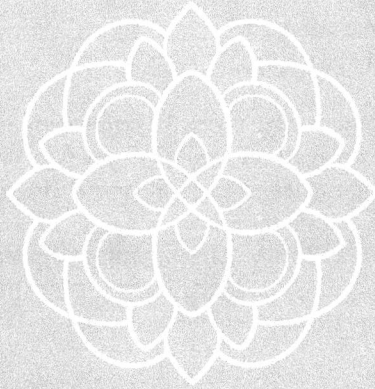

Finding Home

A Path to Emotional
Stability & Self Healing

SECOND EDITION

MAHNAZ JAHANGIRI

Finding Home: A Path to Emotional Stability and Self Healing
SECOND EDITION
Published by Mahnaz Jahangiri
Thousand Oaks, California, U.S.A.

Jahangiri, Mahnaz
Finding Home
Mahnaz Jahangiri

Library of Congress Control Number: 2022911849

ISBN: 979-8-9861592-0-4, 979-8-9861592-3-2 Paperback
ISBN: 979-8-9861592-1-8 Digital

Finding Home Journal: The Companion Guide
ISBN: 979-8-9861592-2-5, 979-8-9861592-4-9 Journal Book

Body, Mind & Spirit > Healing > Prayer & Spiritual
Health & Fitness > Yoga

Photographs by Heirlume Photography.
Book design by Michelle M. White.

QUANTITY PURCHASES:

Schools, companies, professional groups, clubs, and other organizations may
qualify for special terms when ordering quantities of this title.
For information, email info@samadiyoga.com.

Samadi Yoga

"When you lose touch with your inner stillness,
you lose touch with yourself.
When you lose touch with yourself,
you lose yourself in the world."

~ *Eckhart Tolle*

Contents

1. Introduction
Find Your Dharma

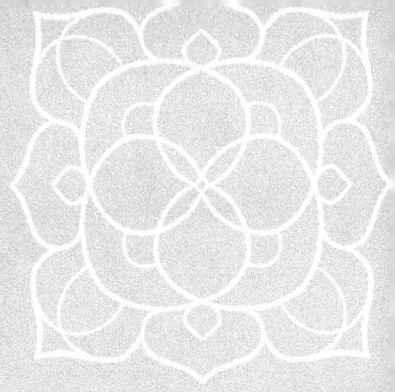

We all have our own story to tell and mine, like so many others, started from my early life experience and basic geography. I slowly became aware of a recurring theme where I felt a sense of not quite belonging. Being born in Tehran, Iran and coming to Los Angeles in 1977 at the age of four was only the beginning. I grew up in the small town of Westlake Village that had very few people who looked like me or who shared the same background. I was in search of finding my home, where I felt I belonged, from early adulthood. My home, the spiritual one, was slowly revealed through my practice of yoga and meditation.

This book serves as a guide for anyone who wants to live a healthier, happier and more present life. A present life where the search for the future and attachment to the past does not take up the full experience, appreciation, and acceptance of the present moment. This book will help set a path for happiness which ultimately resides inside each one of us rather than coming from any outside source. Through a committed practice of yoga and meditation, one can experience a transformation from the inside out and discover where the answers to most challenges lie.

I will cover steps to help create an environment within mind and body that will support proper nurturing, growth, discovery and healing. When these skills are practiced repeatedly on the mat and meditation cushion, these same skills can be used in daily life for self-empowerment, helping ourselves and helping the people around us. This book will help guide you through basic principles of yoga practice in daily life. The yoga practice I refer to, aside from thirty to sixty minutes spent on the mat, also encompasses the practice of life itself. As a guide for new practitioners, this book will also help existing practitioners who need to revisit the basics of yoga philosophy and practice. So, you may ask, how do you become healthier, happier and the best version of yourself?

Invest in yourself with self-reflection, your body with physical yoga practice and your mind with meditation.

FIND YOUR DHARMA

Meditation and yoga help us connect to pure consciousness, where the path to our deepest desires becomes clear. With time and self-reflection, most of us reach a point in our lives where we question our purpose. Through self-observation, we see that mental and behavioral habits lead to patterns in our lives which, if gone unchecked, may repeatedly take us down a dead-end or recurring path.

The path of meditation, yoga and contemplation can help us find our purpose in life. The Sanskrit word Dharma comes from the root "dhri" which means to uplift or uphold. Dharma literally refers to "that which upholds righteousness." A sense of righteousness, of purpose and inspiration, is significant on the spiritual path. The primary quest of a yogi is to discover, follow and live their dharma. The essence of dharma (right action or duty) is doing the right thing and doing it all the time.

Through self-reflection and observation, we learn to take responsibility and understand the power that lies within by recognizing our thoughts, patterns and behaviors.

Meditation and yoga can help us create stillness and connect to ourselves at deeper levels. Even if we don't know the exact details of our ultimate calling, we can tune into what brings us peace through right and conscious action. Right action includes action within ourselves and with the people around us. These right actions are egoless and fully conscious, based on love and goodness that resides within each of us. By having a strong foundational yoga and meditation practice, we can find that purpose. The purpose that will serve others simultaneously will serve ourselves. Hopefully, the purpose and inspiration we find will make us feel fulfilled, at peace and happy throughout our lives.

My personal journey started when I turned to yoga and meditation practice to help manage the daily stresses of work. Once I finished college and began my career, I realized that the stress with television production was going to be an ongoing theme. I knew that I would have to learn how to manage the pressure and turned to yoga and meditation.

Through my practice of yoga, I began to take more ownership over my life, my thoughts and my actions. I let go of my victim mentality and learned to take care of myself at a deeper level. I realized that the situation I found myself in was due to my own actions. The negative results had to do with my unconscious reactions to life events. This daily self-reflection became a self-help tool that moved me out of the victim mentality and into the metaphoric driver's seat. With my steady practice of meditation and yoga, I create the space where I find a connection to my deeper self while simultaneously working through life's daily challenges.

My desire to help others began very early in life. As a child, I don't recall being asked what I wanted to be when I grew up. Yet my earliest thoughts were that I wanted to help people somehow. My parents always had a high respect for doctors, so I thought, "I'll be a doctor!"

The limited belief system in my social environment along with cultural belief systems reinforced that the best paths to choose were to either enter Medical School or Law School. Since I was a fairly strong student scholastically, I decided to major in Biology and aim for Medical School. After two years and several science classes, I began to doubt the choice I had made. Competition was extremely high and I realized that I did not enjoy the sciences beyond Biology and Anatomy.

After a summer away as an au pair in France, I returned home with some clarity and decided to make a different choice. I knew that I no longer wanted to be a medical doctor. Living in Los Angeles, I chose a field that I believed would have unlimited potential, so I decided to change my major to Radio, Television and Film. After 2 more years of University and internships at Sony Studios and MGM Studios, I graduated with my Bachelor of Arts from California State University of Northridge. Although I had no specific direction in the field, I spent ten years in the television Game Show industry. In the midst of my television production career, I found my love for yoga and decided to teach. I found something I truly enjoyed and realized that I may have found my purpose.

I discovered a different path to contributing to humanity while fulfilling my wish to help others. Not only did I find something I loved doing and something that felt right, but I had the satisfaction of seeing the immediate results in the students. Most people come to practice yoga and meditation with some form of pain, whether it be emotional or physical. With a thorough practice, most students experience less pain and more energy, along with a sense of calm and peace. When teaching, I am completely immersed in being present and experience pure awareness. Teaching is like a meditation for me, I am grateful to have the expertise to guide anyone toward better health and ultimately more happiness.

Just like oxygen is necessary for us to breathe, I believe that some form of yoga practice is necessary for us all. Everyone who has a mind and a body can and will benefit from a yoga practice. Everyone who finds challenges in daily life can and will benefit from the practice of yoga. My drive to introduce yoga to all is not just for the physical benefits but, more importantly, for the mental and emotional benefits.

In my first year as a business owner, I offered classes in the original hot yoga style with twenty-six postures and two breathing exercises practiced in a heated yoga room. This style of yoga was considered intimidating and most times discouraging for many people. This was because the heat in the studio often rose above 100 degrees. Back in the 1990s, when I committed to my practice, yoga in a hot room was not as popular as it is today.

Upon opening the first studio, it was important for me to create a space that was welcoming, serene, and not intimidating. The space needed to be safe and clean for students to heal their bodies and minds with the practice of 28 postures.

Knowing that the sequence and the hot room would not be popular amongst all, I made sure to continue my own education to learn the more popular styles of yoga, mainly Vinyasa and guided meditation. As time went on, I created classes and sequences to accommodate everyone, including yoga in an unheated room, yoga for teens, kids, and families and even offered a small number of classes with music. The music was always supportive and calming and fit the mood or style of yoga being taught.

As teachers, educators and community leaders, it is a responsibility to continue to educate oneself and inform others properly. I have always taken this task very seriously. Once I began to introduce a variety of classes, simultaneously I started to organize retreats and shortly thereafter designed my own teacher training program.

To make a commitment to any form of education and teaching, I believe it is important to understand all the details of the field. It is also important to stay updated with the latest research and studies. This responsibility as a teacher and educator was something that I did not take lightly.

When I opened my first studio in 2008, the only training certificate I had achieved was for the Original Hot Yoga from The Ghosh Yoga College of India. This style of yoga was made popular by Bikram Choudhury. Although I had previously explored other styles, at that time I found the greatest results with the 28-pose sequence done in a heated room.

To fully understand the background of this sequence, I wanted to educate myself about the lineage. The Bikram Yoga sequence was derived from the Bishnu Charan Ghosh lineage. Ghosh was Paramahansa Yogananda's younger brother. Yogananda was the author of the most popular yoga novel called *Autobiography of a Yogi*. Bikram Yoga consisted of 28 postures extrapolated from a longer lineage of over 80 poses taught by Bishnu Ghosh.

Along with the Ghosh lineage, I delved into the Krishnamacharya lineage. This lineage has branched into more popular styles of yoga. It also produced notable teachers such as Patabhi Jois who placed Ashtanga Yoga on the map, BKS Iyengar who developed Iyengar Yoga along with Indra Devi, who was one of the few recognized female teachers of her time.

My mission was to offer the best program which suited all practitioners, welcomed every age, body type and included modifications for common and more complex injuries.

I created Samadi Yoga with an intention and a clear understanding of the overall philosophies and histories of the practices. The level of instruction, guidance and care that was reinforced with my instructors was something I was very proud of. This is a quality that is not easily found in many spaces that are now offering yoga.

Our society has reached a point of chronic attention deficit which has driven us to seek immediate gratification in all areas, even with disciplines such as yoga and meditation. The most effective health practices such as yoga and meditation, take practice, determination and repetition. Recent studies have found the United States to be the most "stressed out" country in the world. Now, more than ever, it is imperative that we maintain proper emotional and mental health. Yoga helps to reinforce awareness of the breath, calms the nervous system, strengthens the immune system and helps to maintain proper strength and mobility throughout the body. Consistent practice also counteracts chronic inflammation, which is a precursor to many diseases.

COMMON MYTHS ABOUT YOGA

There are some misconceptions about yoga regarding who may and may not benefit from the physical practice. Yoga is for everyone — anyone who has a mind, body and soul. All human life forms are breathing and thinking beings with physical bodies. The body that we inhabit needs care, attention and maintenance. Whether it be simple breathing techniques or pure sitting meditation, yoga fills these needs. Asana (aa-suh-nuh) is the sanskrit term for yoga postures. Each aspect of yoga has distinct health benefits that mainly cater to spiritual and mental health development, which encompass emotional and physical improvements as well. Yoga benefits health at every level.

Lack of Flexibility

The most common excuse that people resort to when asked why they don't begin a yoga practice is that they lack flexibility. Yoga postures help build more flexibility in the body and more range and movement in the joints. Age, sports, or even inactivity tend to create tightness and weakness in the muscles and restrict proper joint function. A consistent yoga practice will help to alleviate these common problems with reduced tension in the muscles and restored mobility in the joints.

Intimidated to be in a Class

As of March 2020, I began teaching online classes. The Virtual Yoga studio has been a wonderful way for students to join both in the comfort of their own home and to avoid the in-person group classes. The group classes may feel intimidating for new students, yet with more options to practice online, beginners may find it more inviting to try a class and have the teacher demonstrate each pose with step-by-step guidance. To join me online, visit www. samadiyoga.com.

Most well-explained yoga classes consist of both direction and information to help guide you through each and every pose. Yoga takes concentration and focus, which improve with each class. As a beginner in a group class, rest assured that the practice is about focusing on one's own practice and not any other student. In the group setting, new students are usually encouraged to avoid standing in front of the class, so that it would be easier to follow along with more experienced practitioners. This way, the class becomes a lot less intimidating and allows each person to practice at their own pace. A yoga practice should be done regularly, so in no time you will experience more ease in attending online and in-person group classes.

Faithful Practitioners of a Religious Group

Yoga does not have to do with any religion or religious group. Yoga is about connecting to your deeper self by using your breath and body. Even if Sanskrit words are used to give a posture's name or breathing technique, it does not have to do with any religion but with one of the ancient languages of India. The Sanskrit language is seldom to never used anymore. Yoga is about mental observations, movement of the body and ultimately to connect to the higher self. It is not a belief or religious practice.

No Familiarity with Yoga Postures and Sanskrit Names

I recommend that new yoga practitioners find experienced, compassionate and well-educated teachers who explain postures clearly. If Sanskrit words are used, the English translation usually follows. A word you may often hear in various practices is the Sanskrit word, "Namaste". It is equivalent to a thank you and a greeting used either before or after class. The literal translation means "the light in me respects the light in you." Never be embarrassed to ask teachers what they are communicating in class, whether it be about details of the pose or the meaning of any Sanskrit term.

Back Injuries

Yoga is one of the best things to do if you suffer from back injuries. There are numerous causes for back pain, and most back pain is not understood or properly diagnosed. Some people have claimed that yoga hurt their back or triggered an old injury. The problem is not the yoga, but the way that the practice is done.

A simple fact about the human body is that all of us go through deterioration as we age; this includes the structure of the spinal column. Most human bodies will experience slipped discs, bulging discs, or some kind of herniation. Some people with common spinal degenerations go through their lives not ever experiencing pain. Yet deterioration of the spine is best treated by building strong back muscles that protect and support the spine. Through the practice of yoga poses, the spine benefits from full mobility, flexibility and traction to maintain proper space between the vertebrae. A good yoga sequence will always include spine strengthening postures that create stability for the deteriorating spine. It is crucial to practice with awareness so as not to create pain. Yoga practice reinforces listening to the body, and the body communicating with information on how to proceed. If after a yoga practice you experience extreme pain or discomfort, this is an indicator that the practice was approached too aggressively. Keep in mind more is not always better. Practice with awareness, maintaining connection to the breath and feeling the sensations within the body.

Other Injuries

Ongoing practice will soon reveal itself as a form of physical therapy for the body. How? By restoring muscle strength and flexibility, restoring range of motion in the joints and improving overall blood flow and circulation. Any disorder in the body, whether it be structural or internal, is helped with movement and blood flow. The yoga poses help to create a series of compressions so that when released, fresh oxygenated blood flow is brought back to the area. Healing the body takes attention, daily work and reinforcing proper blood flow and circulation. Stagnation and lack of movement creates more pain, inflammation and ultimately disease.

Various Diseases

Yoga practice benefits the muscular and skeletal systems of the body along with the nine other bodily systems. The 11 bodily systems include the circulatory, digestive, endocrine, integumentary (hair, skin, and nails), lymphatic or immune, muscular, nervous, urinary, reproductive, respiratory, and the skeletal systems.

The compression postures have an amazing benefit to the endocrine system and lymphatic systems of the body. The lymphatic or immune system is responsible for fighting illness and disease. The lymph nodes, which are part of the lympthatic system, are spread throughout the body. Most of the nodes tend to cluster around the neck, the chest and armpits and the groin. All the postures that effect these areas will create a stretch or compression which helps to move the lymph fluid. The lymph nodes contain immune cells that help fight infection by attacking and destroying the germs that are carried in through the lymph fluid. For example, back bends will stretch around the throat, chest, armpits and the groin, which benefits the major clusters of lymph nodes and facilitates the capability of fighting various diseases.

Overweight or Underweight

Another common excuse for avoiding a yoga practice is the opinion of being too plump or too slim. As mentioned earlier, yoga poses help balance all systems of the body including the endocrine system, or hormone balancing system. The thyroid gland, which is part of the endocrine system, releases hormones and controls metabolism. Yoga postures create compressions to endocrine glands which are in the head, throat and lower back. The thyroid and parathyroid glands are in the throat, while the kidneys, located in the lower back, are part of the endocrine system. Most yoga postures have some effect on the neck and throat as well as the lower back, whether through a stretch, compression or a twist. Compressions and stretching create blood flow to these glands to help with the overall balance of hormone levels.

The stress hormone cortisol may affect the abdominal area of the body. This is the most common area that accumulates fat due to long-term stress. Many practitioners notice reduced abdominal fat because of the stress-reducing benefits of a regular practice.

On the flip side, I have worked with numerous students dealing with low body weight and even anorexia. They, too, have seen results both in the balance of hormones and more importantly in negative thinking patterns. A consistent yoga practice ultimately helps us reconnect and appreciate our body. When there is a stronger connection within ourselves, there tends to be more self-acceptance and self-love.

Vegan and Vegetarian

Choosing a vegan or vegetarian diet is not a prerequisite to practice yoga and meditation. Although limiting and abstaining from animal meat results in more joint mobility, the lack of enough protein can cause weakness in the muscles. If you choose to abstain from animal proteins, be sure to educate yourself on healthier alternatives.

One of the eight limbs of the Yoga Sutras is non-violence. This pertains to any killing of living creatures and even of violent thoughts or behaviors. Another component of yoga practice is non-judgment. As a practitioner, it's helpful to not only accept ourselves, but also all people around us. Each of us as individuals will find what works for us through trial and error. We benefit by having our individuality, observing our own bodies and learning to make choices without subscribing to a collective belief system.

What works for one person may not work for another. It is important to discover what works for you and your own body. The best way to understand how certain foods affect your body and mind is to become aware of the energy, strength and mental clarity that result with different choices. A consistent practice will help you tune in to your body daily to determine this. For example, the result of alcohol consumption is usually a feeling of lower energy. When consuming foods that are fried or heavy, you may feel the discomfort in the body and belly. On the other hand, if you don't consume enough food, you may notice weakness, lack of strength and dizziness. Experiment with different foods. Try to maintain a healthy balance of fresh fruits, vegetables, nuts and protein. Most importantly, let your body be your guide.

Marijuana and Drug Use

This may be disappointing to some readers but being high and taking yoga do not fit or complement one another. Neither do past trends in yoga practice such as beer and yoga, wine and yoga or weed and yoga. Yoga and meditation are meant to be practiced with a clear mind to help create more focus and discipline. Some practitioners may be on prescribed medications, but if a medication alters mental clarity and stability, it is important to practice with care. Avoid taking over-the-counter medications such as ibuprofen or acetaminophen before practice. It is important to listen and feel the pain in the body with full attention as opposed to dulling or numbing the sensations. Some may think that it is easier to practice with less pain from an injury, yet the downside is that you may not understand what is happening in the body and the dulling prevents sensations that may tell you to back off. Yoga and meditation are about awareness, connection, and consciousness. Yoga will create calm in the body and will result in a natural high that you may have never felt before!

Age: Too Old or too Young

You are never too old or too young to practice yoga. I began teaching my father when he was in his late seventies, and I have fellow teachers who have parents and students start a practice well into their eighties. Depending on limitations and energy levels, the option of using a yoga chair is useful and effective for many poses.

Babies are natural practitioners on both physical and mental levels. Many of us have witnessed an infant performing a perfect Happy Baby Pose laying on their back and grabbing their feet! On the mental level, the early years of human life tend to be more in the present moment. As we age and accumulate more experience, we tend to lose the ability to stay present. We get lost in obsessive thinking, worrying and judging.

I have taught five-year-olds both in-studio and at local elementary schools. The kids ages ranged from five to eleven years old. Luckily today, many kids are being introduced to yoga and meditation to help with focus, concentration, and coordination. Yoga practice as a way to build physical and mental discipline can be taught to most kids effectively from the ages of five and up.

If you are interested in living a healthier, happier, balanced, connected and pain-free life, try all your options in meditation and yoga. Experiment with different styles and find what methods work for you. At the end of this book, I have outlined a simple sequence that will guide you through a safe and effective practice. Try it at least three days a week for four weeks and enjoy the results in body and mind.

2. Finding Home
A Place or a Feeling?

"...You realize that all along there was something tremendous within you, and you did not know it."
~ *Paramahansa Yogananda*

The word home usually represents a physical location or a space. I was born in the city of Tehran in the country of Iran. When my parents came to Los Angeles in the summer of 1977, they were still undecided as to where the future of their children would land. The choices were to start a new life here in the United States or to return to an unstable political situation in Iran.

I grew up in Southern California and visited Iran 20 years later at the age of 24. Although I had few vague memories of the home we lived in, I felt I was a foreigner in the country where I was born. This was apparent to the Iranians because of the way I held myself and simply by the way I walked. Emotionally and mentally, I felt like a visitor. Throughout the trip I experienced some flashbacks that resembled vague and unclear dreams. My discomfort and feeling of not belonging did not make complete sense to me at the time.

Most of us grasp onto a physical location such as a home or even a country to represent where we belong. Our social and survival conditioning is to someday create a home, and ultimately a family. Unfortunately we are not taught early in life that home needs to be created within ourselves. Creating a home within ourselves means connecting to the sense of self at a deeper level, including having self-love, self-compassion and ultimately self-acceptance. Once we learn to create a loving environment within ourselves, then it becomes much easier to find the home and loving environment wherever we choose to live and settle down.

As social beings, we need love, and we thrive in having a sense of community and a sense of belonging. Research studies prove that socializing helps prolong our lives. What is important to know is that our social circles and support systems are more important than our physical location. As human beings, we collectively bond and do great things together. We have moved through the ages with combined inventions and made large steps with support systems and fellow contributors. Our communities and collaborations move us forward with shared energy and common interest.

Where we find love and stability is fundamentally created in our emotional development. We, as humans, can and do adapt to any situation. Food, shelter and love are the basic necessities, yet the most important home is in our own mind and body.

Creating stability starts within ourselves. This can be reinforced with a consistent practice of meditation which creates calm within. The calm is created by slowing down and observing the thoughts which in turn helps us create emotional stability. When our thoughts are attached to future or past thinking, we tend to be in a state of sadness, anxiety, panic and even depression. From a stable emotional place, we can make the right decisions and choices with awareness and clarity.

Our thinking patterns become our stories which can be reinforced through our lives unconsciously. It is important to embrace that our thoughts are not necessarily the truth. Our thoughts are just an idea of what we believe is true at any given moment in time.

Years ago, I mentioned this in class and afterwards a student approached me with such awe. This was a brand-new concept she had been introduced to. She mentioned, "I never thought for a moment that my thoughts could be untrue!" I could sense that she had realized something that would give her a little more peace and relief by not taking her thoughts so seriously.

Our thoughts can help create our reality, but once we allow our thoughts to come and go, we can let go of the grasp we have and avoid attaching so intently. This alone ultimately makes the thought less powerful. Thoughts are just concepts we tend to believe at a moment in time. Yoga and meditation can help us become aware of the thoughts that create tension and negativity. The practice helps teach us to simply notice our own mental patterns. The mental patterns and cyclical thinking take us out of the present moment. These patterns often turn into judgments, doubts, internal conflict and suffering.

One of my favorite books, *The Four Agreements*, by Don Miguel Ruiz, highlights four guidelines to living a happier life. The agreements are to be impeccable with your word, don't take anything personally, don't make assumptions and always do your best. The one that helps me the most is to try to not take anything personally. Each individual has their own thought process based on experiences, culture, personality and development. We don't really know what someone is thinking and how their thought process has evolved. We are all struggling and finding our own peace and place in life. As long as we are in the process of life, there is or will be at some point a challenge to work through. Ultimately, we have no control over what comes up in our lives, but we can develop skills to help with resilience, mental and emotional health and learning to be present.

Yoga as therapy for pain and inflammation in the body is secondary to the mental health benefits of practicing presence, self-reflection, and centering oneself. Detaching from the cyclical thought patterns, even if it's for only a moment, is key. This is the beauty of meditation. To learn to connect to the deeper or higher self by learning to be in the now. The deeper or higher self is unchanging based on external circumstances such as time, money or any concept. The deeper or higher self is the witnessing presence which always resides in the background.

A meditation or yoga practice can be compared to a good night's sleep. Rest gives us a break from our thinking minds, allows the nervous system to calm and allows the body to do its repairs by decreasing inflammation. Meditation helps us do this "repair work" for the body and mind but in an awake state. With meditation, by observing our thoughts and reconnecting to our deeper self, we find home. Our body feels better with less tension and we find the peace that is always there waiting for us. With meditation we learn to rest into our home, into our bodies, and to settle back into a calm and peaceful place.

BUILDING HEALTHY HABITS

To feel at home in our own mind and body, below is an outline highlighting three basic areas for optimal physical, mental and emotional health.

On the physical level, positive health habits begin by taking steps to include the following in our daily lives: 1. Meditation and yoga practice 2. Eating well and drinking plenty of water 3. Getting enough sleep.

Daily Meditation and Yoga Practice

Unlike a typical physical exercise such as weightlifting, yoga can be practiced daily and meditation can be practiced hourly. We can slowly begin to incorporate a meditative quality to our daily tasks. For example, as we make our morning coffee or tea, pay attention to the breathing and simultaneously focus on the task being done. Meditation does not necessarily need to be done seated or on a cushion with the eyes closed. Meditation can be done during daily activities with awareness of the breath, noticing bodily sensations and letting go of unnecessary thinking.

Physical yoga can work from the outside in, whereas meditation works from the inside out. Most people have a more challenging time sitting still as opposed to moving physically in space. Most may know and agree, it all begins and ends in the mind. For most of us, battling our "monkey" minds, we tend to do better with physical movement which captures our attention. This seems to be less daunting than to sit and observe the mind. This is why the physical practice of Hatha Yoga began 1,000 years ago, to prepare the mind for the more challenging Meditation practices that started about 5,000 years ago. For many people, it is more attainable to move the body and calm the mind to get ready for meditation than the other way around.

Hydration and Nutrition

Most people are dehydrated. If you consume the minimum amount of water necessary per day, you will most likely notice immediate results. An easy way to measure this is to drink half your body weight in ounces. For example, if your bodyweight is 100 pounds, you should be drinking fifty ounces of water a day. There are eight ounces in one cup. If you have a daily diet that includes caffeine and/or alcohol, it is necessary to drink at least one extra cup of water. Caffeine and alcohol are diuretics, meaning they drain the body of fluids and cause increased urination. Keep in mind the human adult body is made up of "up to 60 percent water," according to H.H. Mitchell, Journal of Biological Chemistry. "The brain and heart are composed of 73 percent water, and the lungs are about 83 percent water." So, clearly, we need water for the brain and the lungs for all systems to perform properly. The lack of water causes improper brain function which controls all aspects of the body. So be sure to drink the minimum daily ounces of water each day to allow the body to do what it needs.

Proper nutrition is also a major ingredient for health and wellness. How do you determine the effects of health with food? First, notice how you feel after a heavy meal as opposed to how you feel when you eat lighter and balanced meals that include vegetables and protein. As you become more sensitive to the effects of foods you consume, you may also notice fluctuations in mood. You may observe that junk food usually makes you feel unenergized — heavy, dull, foggy-brained and moody. In contrast, make note of how you feel after a healthy and light meal. You will most likely feel more energy and clearer mentally. The sensations and moods you experience are the result of the effects on hormones. Hormone balance and imbalance effect our emotional and mental states.

Proper nutrition helps to keep blood sugar levels and hormone levels balanced. The two are interrelated and these two have a direct effect on mood. Food can be used as medicine to help the body along with the emotional and mental state. When the body receives the necessary nutrients, there is decreased inflammation and usually less discomfort in the body. When the body is in pain or in poor health, it can serve as a distraction. This distraction makes it more challenging to sit still comfortably, to focus the mind, connect to the breath, and ultimately to connect to the deeper self.

A common question that comes up is what to eat, and what I personally eat to stay healthy and vibrant. My answer usually is the same which is that everyone is different. Just because one practices yoga and meditation does not mean that a commitment needs to be made to be vegetarian or vegan. I believe it is important to care for our body at the same time to care for the planet. One is directly related to the other. We are all connected and what we do has an immediate effect on everything around us.

Everyone must determine for themselves which foods help them feel their best. Energy, strength, balance and nourishment are the key components. A physical yoga practice will help determine this. Part of a consistent yoga practice is the acknowledgement of the varying energy levels in the body day-to-day. Through yoga you will begin to notice the difference in the strength of the muscles and the flexibility in the joints. You may also become more sensitive to inflammation and bloating within your body and especially in the gut. Inflammation, weakness and imbalance will become obvious while observing the body through various yoga postures. Tuning into your body will help you determine what the body needs and how it reacts to different foods and nutrients.

Sleep

Getting sufficient sleep every night is essential for each of us, but exactly how much varies by person. As infants and teenagers, we tend to need more sleep, yet as we age and move into our Golden Years we tend to need less. The general recommendation is six to eight or nine hours of sleep per night. It is important to be consistent with your bedtime. Try to be disciplined with the time the lights are turned off (with no smartphones or iPads) and with the time you wake up each day. To determine the necessary amount for you, take note of your energy level and mental clarity throughout the day.

If your schedule permits, short naps help keep the energy stable and the mind fresh. This is a good way to rely less on caffeine and sugar to get you through the late morning or afternoon slump. Caffeine will give you a short burst of energy but the fatigue that follows may be worse. The body and, more specifically, the hormone levels will waiver to rebalance.

Sugar is another ingredient we overuse to increase energy. This has more negative effects than positive ones. Choose wisely by sticking to natural sugars, such as fruit and, if necessary, dried fruit as opposed to candy and processed foods.

Another option to increase energy is to take five minutes to work on diaphragmatic breathing, kapalabhati breathing or alternate nostril breathing. I will cover these techniques at the end of the book before introducing the sequence of postures. The goal is to keep the body in balance without using outside stimulants.

Protein bars are a big trend; it's astounding that protein bars can take up entire aisles of many health food markets. Read the labels and make note of the ingredients that you don't recognize. If you don't know what it is, don't eat it. A general rule of thumb for healthy eating: avoid foods that are packaged and processed. Include fresh foods consisting of fruits, vegetables and nuts.

EMOTIONAL HEALTH

Self-Worth

All through our lives we tackle issues based on our self-worth. It is usually buried beneath our biggest challenges and frustrations. The value we learn to reflect within ourselves begins in childhood and continues until our death. We process life from our interactions and relationships growing up. The relationships start with our parents and continue with grandparents, siblings, teachers, employers, friends and lovers. The positive and negative effects of these early relationships continue into adulthood. Many of our triggers through our lives may be connected to self-worth and show up as events that we tend to struggle with.

To evaluate self-worth issues, it is important to let go of old and limiting beliefs. These old belief systems are stories that are not true. These stories perpetuate through media and social media, advertising and even pop culture. Much of the world falsely believes that self-worth is connected to net worth. This belief system keeps us detached from the deeper self and keeps us stuck in the outside, superficial world. If we lose our power and our control over ourselves, we become easier targets to manipulate. If there is low self-worth or the belief that there is something lacking, then it's easier to reach for an idea or material object to fulfill that void. When we feel empowered and connected within ourselves, it becomes more challenging for anyone or anything to manipulate and control us for personal gain.

Through meditation, yoga and self-reflection, we learn to delve into our worth and potential at the deepest levels. No amount of money or success can determine our true value. We are all part of one consciousness that is beyond any concept. Self-worth begins and ends with us, to know that we are more than our physical body, our life situation or any concept. Spiritual practice helps us connect deeper so that we do not rely on others to determine what we think of ourselves.

When we conduct our lives with an attitude of service and care for others, in addition to self-reflection and therapy, we feel more connected to each other. We have control over very few things, but our own positive thought process is a habit we can build.

Positive thinking and taking care of ourselves with love and nurturing will lead us to the best version of self. We can continue to find happiness by taking responsibility for ourselves and reflecting on our belief system through self-observations and therapy, yoga and meditation. When we take responsibility for our mental, emotional and physical health, we have more influence over the direction of our lives.

Reinforcement of our self-worth through self-reflection helps guide us down the path of self-respect. This self-respect and self-love spreads to the people around us. How we behave towards others has much to do with how we treat ourselves.

There are times where negative situations arise in our lives, but through care and compassion we can create space for ourselves even if it means to remove ourselves completely from the situation. Space allows us to deal with our challenges from a less reactive and clearer perspective.

My meditation and yoga practice helps me to move through challenging situations and to accept that most suffering is tied to thoughts and experiences that are all fleeting and changing.

Many books on yoga, philosophy and spirituality highlight the fact that happiness can be found in helping to bring it to others. As teachers, educators, counselors or coaches, the foundation of the work rests in service. The main purpose of the work is to serve and be of service to others.

Some of the most satisfied people you meet in life are the ones who feel that they have a purpose and usually are of service to others. A life of purpose is a life well-lived. The choice to serve others helps with better health on an emotional and mental level. When we make someone else happy or help to nourish them with attention, listening, love or even food, we tend to be happier within ourselves.

Competition

Competition, if gone unobserved, can be directly related to self-worth. Self-worth is not something that is attained or accumulated but something that is understood and felt. Competition is a repetitious game of proving self-worth. Outside of sporting competitions, notice the behaviors in yourself that cause you to compare and compete with others. This may seem positive in small instances yet over time you realize it's a losing battle with one-self.

For someone who may be working through insecurities, every situation becomes a challenge. Underneath many of our struggles, the battle of self-acceptance may be at the root. Notice when these moments arise. You may find that it creates much of the internal and physical tension experienced.

To help create connection, self-love, self-acceptance and even self-worth, begin a simple morning practice by looking in the mirror and telling yourself that you love you. If you find this to be too much of a challenge, think of someone in your life who loves you. If that's too hard, at least tell yourself that you see you. You may also imagine yourself as a young child or even imagine your future, wiser self. The most important part of this practice is to do it often and to really mean it. A good therapist can also help navigate complexities that cover up our challenge with self-love and self-acceptance.

Another way to discover self-love is to give love to others. Do your best to love yourself and treat others the way you want to be treated. If you want affirmation, give affirmation; if you want love, give love; if you want attention, give attention. If you don't believe you are doing your best now, then practice more awareness and less reaction. Create space to reflect and incorporate some form of reflection. Options that may help can be journaling, finding a good therapist or participating in group therapy or counseling.

Only we know what the mental activity consists of. We can practice ending the patterns of abusive self-talk. We don't need to endlessly search for positive affirmations. The first step is to simply notice the thoughts. This is what meditation teaches; awareness of our thoughts and space to reflect and ultimately let go.

Researchers can see the effects of meditation on brain scans. The amygdala is the area of the brain that governs emotion, fear, and stress response. Research has proven that meditation helps lower reactivity and promote recovery more quickly after a stressful event occurs. Although our survival instinct is to compete, it's important to become aware of the equal worth that we all have as humans. Incorporating meditation will help you discover a way to find inner peace, self- acceptance and self-love.

Surrender

Practicing surrender is a recurrent theme with meditation and yoga. To transition from a place of resistance to a space of acceptance is the way to tune into the present moment. Practice not labeling or judging the present moment but allowing it to be. This practice can be done at any moment in your day, especially when you notice struggle and dissatisfaction.

For any creative process to flow, the mind needs to be focused and clear, which means the nervous system needs to be calm. When there is high stress or anxiety, the nervous system is in fight-or-flight mode. The mind is not functioning at its full-potential because the bodily systems are designed to take over and keep us alive. The nervous system gets triggered to get you out of danger and get you to safety. These effects include increased heart rate, shorter breathing and tightening in the hip flexors. When the breath is short and the heart rate is up, it becomes impossible to be in a creative zone.

Meditation and yoga reinforce guiding the mind and body towards a calm and restorative mode for our nervous system. Through our practice, the feeling of home can be compared to a calm state of mind. Distractions, stories, negative feedback and fear not only keep us in fight-or-flight mode but keep us from finding our home that exists within ourselves.

Food, shelter and love are the basic necessities for all humans. Learn to give your mind the good food of positive thinking. Shelter yourself from negativity, harm and self-abuse, and give your body and yourself love to function optimally. Focus more on the inside and less on the outside. Yoga and meditation will guide us back to our deeper selves and unite us in our common humanity and ultimately to consciousness.

HOME AND SAFETY

Feeling safe in the space we inhabit is very important. A safe structure is a place where we are warm and protected, free from natural and man-made dangers. Feeling emotional safety is just as important to the physical safety in our space. For us to live a healthy and balanced life, let's consider how our nervous system is affected.

Yoga practice has been popularized mostly on the physical benefits such as greater flexibility and strength. The aspect that is now being highlighted is the calming effect to the nervous system, along with the benefits on emotional and mental health. Our culture and society are moving faster, introducing us to new technology and feeding us an overwhelming amount of information. This is impacting kids and young adults in negative ways.

Progress is usually good and cannot be stopped, but how we handle ourselves in our current environment is crucial. Artificial intelligence is a larger part of our society, but we need to stay ahead of technology. We need to be cognizant and keep technology from taking over our individual thinking.

Be very aware of technology and its ability to take over our thinking capacity. It is important for us to check in with ourselves and consider how we make our personal choices. It is important to be sure that we are not making choices based on an algorithm that benefits a company's bottom line.

The advancement of technology, bombardment of information and other distractions is negatively affecting our youth with higher levels of anxiety and depression. The most important home we have is the one in our minds and bodies. To create a safe home in our minds and in our bodies, we need to reinforce positive habits that elevate us mentally, emotionally and physically.

Some things to consider would be, what is the physical space I live in and do I feel safe? How can I create a safe environment for myself? Is the nervous system calm in this space? What can I do to heal, calm and nurture myself?

Make it a habit to take a day, half a day, or at least several hours each week to detach from smartphones, smartwatches, laptops and other devices. Schedule time to turn off all external distractions. Experience the freedom you create by eliminating the external noise.

Our long-term survival as a human species depends not only on our planet but our ability to connect to ourselves daily on a deeper level. To find our own truth means to connect to our deeper self and to wake up from unconscious behaviors and actions. Yoga, meditation, nature and spiritual practice help to keep us connected.

3. Samadhi
The 8th Limb of Yoga

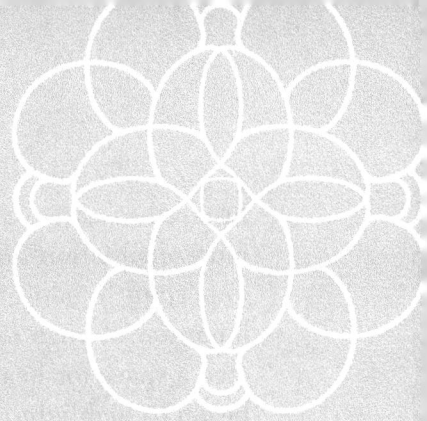

"The primary cause of unhappiness is never the situation
but your thoughts about it."
~*Eckhart Tolle*

For the first time in my life, I embraced the true essence of Samadhi through a ten-day Vipassana meditation course in Twentynine Palms, California. Samadhi means concentration and mastery of the mind through meditation.

Samadhi is the eighth limb of Patanjali's Yoga Sutras[1] and the final stage of self-realization, further outlined in Chapter 6. Patanjali was one of the first to define yoga philosophy in a written format.

The course involves ten full days of meditation starting at 4:30 a.m. and ending with a 9 p.m. video lecture from Master Vipassana Teacher, Goenka. The day includes a breakfast hour, lunch hour and an afternoon tea, each followed by a break with the option of a contemplative walk.

The training had such a profound impact that it led me to rename my yoga program and studio to Samadi Yoga. At that point I decided to incorporate the most important element of yoga practice, the practice of meditation. With the new name, I was

---

1 Patanjali's Yoga Sutras is the most recognized yoga philosophy text and writings. There has been much research as to whether Patanjali was one person or a group of writers who compiled the famous texts.

inspired to create a more inclusive yoga program and introduce more meditation and yoga philosophy to the community. It was important to educate the community I was serving with the full intention of yoga as meditation and mastery of the mind. I created a space for healing beyond the physical level of practice and began to highlight the mental disciplines.

Liberation from mental and emotional pain is reinforced in the meditation practice whereas liberation from physical pain is reinforced in physical yoga practice. Many times, the pain can be interrelated. The seven limbs preceding Samadhi create a path toward the optimal destination which is a sense of home both in our minds and bodies.

Prior to going to the course, I was feeling sad and lost due to a relationship that had ended. I felt deflated, finding myself with the familiar sense of emptiness. I knew that my perspective and approach had to be changed. I was clearly looking outside of myself for love and happiness. The message that I received during the retreat was that the love I was searching for had to be love for myself. The happiness I was searching for was always deep inside. I realized the story of finding happiness within someone else was a perspective that needed to be changed.

I personally like to use the word peace in place of happiness. Happiness is too simple and fleeting. Yet peace is deep and steady and can be reinforced with the practice of connectedness and meditation.

The path of insight, awareness and enlightenment helps us discover that when our minds are calm and our actions loving, we discover better overall health. Life flows better and feels better. This balance of awareness practice and healthy habits helps take us through our lives with a little more ease and a little less suffering.

Anicha is a Sanskrit[2] word that means change. Life is constantly changing, and we are in an ongoing momentum of transitions. Some are more uncomfortable than others. Life will continue to challenge us and guide us to different paths. We are better served if we allow the natural flow to take place, to adapt without resistance and to train ourselves mentally with meditation. There is an automatic and reactive tendency to resist change within many of us. Unfortunately, this creates more suffering and possibly prolongs the discomfort of any situation. Our unconscious habit is to try to control all details of our lives with the idea of a specific outcome. We usually believe a specific outcome will give us inner peace. This is another illusion. We cannot control most things in life. The inner peace resides in the practice of letting go. Letting go means learning to surrender to a desired outcome and to live in the moment. Yoga and meditation practice teaches us to accept reality as it is. Meditation also helps train the mind to let go. The practice of letting go becomes crucial in handling life's challenges. The less we try to control, the more we can be in the moment with presence, awareness, and acceptance. This practice helps us experience life with not only less resistance, but also less struggle and less fear.

The state of fear is only conducive when we are in imminent danger. Most of our lives are not spent in situations where there is real danger. Most of our fear is mind-made and lies at the root of our worries, doubts and overall stress.

Our thoughts are what create the danger, and our physiology responds. The physical body does not differentiate between mind-made danger and real, imminent danger. The body will respond to each the same. The heart rate speeds up, the breath becomes short and shallow, the body becomes tense (including the hip flexors, to prepare the body to run) and all the body's systems prepare to get out of harm's way. Ultimately the body is

---

2 Sanskrit is an ancient language of India that is rarely used but recognized due to its origins in Hinduism and Buddhism. Many yoga postures are still referred to by their Sanskrit name.

designed to respond in short spurts, but if the stress and fear modes continue, the immune system becomes weak, and our body is in dis-EASE. This disease will lead to the downward spiral of illness and early death.

The human brain is so complex that scientific studies have yet to fully understand its endless capabilities. Most humans only use a small fraction of their brains daily.

Presence is more a feeling and less a thought. With meditation practice, we train ourselves to observe our thoughts as opposed to becoming our thoughts. Meditation helps create space to pay attention to the breath, to sense the body and to stay rooted in the present moment. The present moment is where we can feel the witnessing presence, the soul, consciousness.

The common experience among people new to meditation is the fluctuation of the mind between past and future events. Presence of mind is when we are completely in the experience of what is happening now. Some questions to ask are How am I breathing? Is my body tense? Usually, the tension is related to a thought about the past or future. Unfortunately, much of our past and future thinking is fear-based. Past thinking is about attaching to events that have happened and not being able to let go. Also, much of future thinking may be linked to fear of the unknown. We think if we can plan, then there will be no surprises. This past and future thinking takes us back to the cycle of being in a constant state of fear and anxiety or sadness. This affects us by causing stress hormones to be released, breathing then suffers and ultimately weakness develops in the immune system. The weakened immune system gives room for illness and virus to settle into the body. The mental virus of thinking becomes more dangerous than the physical virus.

Being means to be present with the current experience. When practicing presence, we are fully conscious. When we are conscious, we are not likely to respond from our subconscious or even unconscious state. The subconscious and unconscious thoughts are what we develop throughout our lives, based on experiences, pains, results and reactivity.

We have all experienced having a conversation with someone who is not fully present or listening. They are planning on what they will be saying next as opposed to attentively listening to the words coming out of our mouth. Many of us can also relate to being in a conversation where we are the one who is lost in thought and not understanding what someone is trying to communicate. This is an example of not being present or conscious in daily interactions. Our minds are too busy thinking and ultimately missing what is happening in front of us in any given moment.

This is part of why it is so important to practice stillness and meditation. In meditation, we train the mind to become comfortable with sitting in stillness and sensing our bodies. The sensing can be compared to listening. To allow for the next moment to unfold. As we learn to observe our body sensations, we create space and notice the mental noise. This practice reinforces our awareness which will in turn help us become attuned to ourselves, along with other people and the world around us.

The best physical yoga practice I ever had was the first class I had taken the day after my ten-day Vipassana course. My mind was focused and quiet, and I was completely in the moment and tuned into my body. Mind and body functioned as one with effortless ease. This experience fortified the goal of yoga practice to discipline the overactive mind and reconnect to the deeper self.

This experience was all I needed to increase the implementation of meditation practice. Unfortunately, a physical practice without the reinforcement of meditation becomes just another workout.

At the start of a yoga practice, either physical or sitting meditation, focusing the mind is a challenge because of the mind's constant fluctuations. With a consistent and disciplined practice, usually halfway through, the thoughts begin to quiet down and subside. By the conclusion of your practice, you will notice the calmness in the mind and body, the connection to the deeper self and the beauty of the yoga practice. The practice of yoga helps us maintain the sense of peace we crave.

An effective practice begins and ends with the focus on the breath, whether it be breath control or breath observation. The way to breathe properly is to inhale and exhale through the nose. If you feel you are struggling to do this, or have any congestion, know that it is ok to open the mouth to assist breathing. Nose breathing has a direct effect on deep breathing which in turn affects the nervous system. Deep breathing helps to calm the nervous system. When the nervous system begins to calm, the body has a chance to restore. Yoga is one of the few physical forms of exercise that restores and reenergizes the body rather than depleting it of energy. This can be tested with just five to ten minutes of meditation. Simply sit with eyes closed or lowered and focus on the flow of the breath. The flow of the breath can be observed with the rise and fall of the chest or belly (or both) and it can also be observed by sensing the breath against the upper lip. If neither of these work, you may even try visualizing an imaginary triangle around the nose and mouth and simply notice the breath moving in and out of the imaginary triangle.

Yoga practice will not only bring the body back to proper functioning but calms the nervous system and clears the mind. When the mind is clear, we can feel our natural state. Throughout my 30-year practice of yoga, I have been grateful for having the tools to help me with challenges. These times of challenge were accompanied with much fear and anxiety. Due to my consistent practice, I made it through each challenge with grace and grit and usually found myself in a healthier place. The practice helps move us through challenges with connection, awareness and calm. I cannot imagine how much more suffering I would endure without the release and the safety that yoga and meditation practice offer me. For me, yoga has been my ultimate guide to finding home.

4. Meditation

The Essential Component of Yoga

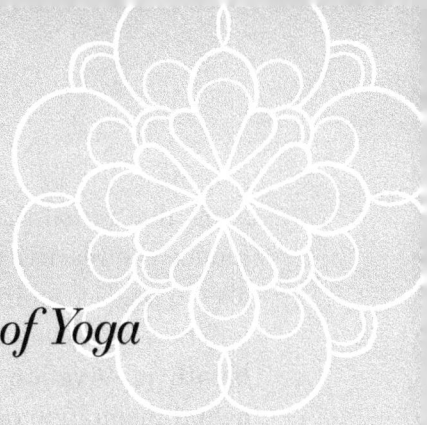

"Being must be felt. It can't be thought."

~ *Eckhart Tolle, "The Power of Now"*

According to the Buddhist philosophy, life is full of suffering, and the way to eliminate suffering is through cessation of mental attachment and resistance.

HOW TO END SUFFERING

Life will throw many challenges our way and we have no control over how, when and to what degree. The amount of suffering can be reduced with our ability to control the mind's reactive tendencies. We can help the reactivity by staying present and grounded, and allowing the challenges to come and learning to let them go. All things in life are in a process of constant change and of coming and going.

The most effective way to discipline the mind is to meditate regularly. Meditation is not the absence of thought; it is the active observation of thought without analysis. Disciplined meditation practice helps to train the brain not to react to situations in a negative, cyclical or automatic ways. The area of the brain which governs the stress response, emotion, fear and fight-or-flight is called the amygdala. Researchers have observed human brains with brain scans that reveal that just 10 continuous sessions help to not only reduce the reactivity in this area during upsetting situations, but also to recover more quickly after a stressful event occurs.

There are several ways to meditate. The various forms include breath observation, candlelight meditation, chanting, transcendental meditation or TM, and the body scan technique.

My preferred method is Vipassana. Vipassana is a Pali, the spoken language of Buddha, word that means to observe things as they really are rather than how they appear to be. The Vipassana meditation is a combination of breath observation and body scan technique. The method begins with Anapana breathing which is breath observation while simultaneously going through the body with a complete scan from head to toes and then back up the body. In the process, neural pathways are created that help sense the body more closely, rooting you in the present moment and removing you from the overactive thinking mind that is not usually in the present moment. The body scan is intended to train the mind to be in a state of awareness by observing sensations, such as cold, heat, tingling, pressure or possibly the lack of any sensation. In the process, you reprogram the brain and bring yourself to present moment experiences rather than mind-made ones. The training guides you to acknowledge sensations through each specific area of the body and to learn to move on to the next area without clinging to or resisting whatever the sensation may be. This process helps to program the brain to respond in the same way to real-life experiences as it does to the experience of "observing and letting go" in meditation practice. The suffering in daily life usually comes from resisting or clinging to things, people, or events.

The training for Vipassana is a ten-day course of silent observation of oneself through this method of meditation. Each full day of meditation is followed by a talk from Goenke, who was the primary teacher of the method. Per Vipassana literature, it is claimed that the vipassana method of meditation was used long before the time of Buddha, yet Buddha initiated the re-introduction of this method.

During the course, the requirements are to abstain from talking, reading and writing. This allows the mind to process information with no other outlet. This way you can get to the root of your individual mental process without external stimulation or distraction. A common day during the course begins at 4:30 a.m. and ends in the evening after a 9 p.m. talk from lead teacher Goenke. His recorded talks cover a variety of topics that help summarize yoga philosophy along with other principles to lead a happier life and a life with less suffering.

The key to starting any meditation practice is to begin with the focus on the breath. The goal is to stay connected and observant of the breath throughout the practice. The breath is directly connected to the nervous system and ultimately to all systems of the body through the brain. The nervous system has two main segments, the central nervous system and the peripheral nervous system. The central nervous system is made up of the brain and spinal cord. The peripheral nervous system is made up of nerves that branch off from the spinal cord and extend to all parts of the body.

The peripheral nervous system is further subdivided into the somatic and the autonomic nervous system.

The somatic nervous system is the part of the peripheral nervous system that handles voluntary control of body movements via skeletal muscles, while the autonomic nervous system acts as an involuntary control system of the body.

The autonomic nervous system is also divided into the sympathetic and the parasympathetic. The sympathetic is the fight-or-flight response and reacts to events that are perceived as stressful, while the parasympathetic is the calming and restoring response. The parasympathetic nervous system decreases respiration and heart rate and increases digestion.

For many of us, our lives are spent in survival mode which is associated with the "fight or flight" or stress-related mode. Adrenaline is released during times of stress or excitement. Adrenaline increases the heart rate, elevates the blood pressure and boosts energy supplies. Cortisol is the primary stress hormone which increases sugar in the bloodstream. Increased cortisol levels lead to the belly fat that appears after extended struggles with stress factors. Optimal health entails the balance of mind and body, encompassing mental, emotional and physical health. Activities such as yoga and meditation help the nervous system function in the calm and restorative mode and less in the fight -or -flight and danger mode.

During times of increased stress, the body releases cortisol, which signals the body of danger. The muscles tense up, the mouth gets dry, the heart rate increases, and breath becomes short and labored. The body immediately prepares to get out of harm's way. Chronic high levels of cortisol prevent the mind from thinking clearly. Hypothetically, if we were to be running away from a dangerous animal or event, we need our body to act quicker than the mind, otherwise we would be eliminated. In moments of high-stress and danger, it is detrimental, and most likely impossible, for the creative mind to get out of harm's way. The body is in overdrive and the survival instinct takes over. Once the nervous system is calm, the body restores, the mind functions clearly and we can continue with caution and awareness.

Notice your breath and heart rate next time you are upset or stressed. If the tension is released with a good cry, the body's natural function takes over with deep breaths to calm the nervous system.

Vipassana meditation is a practice of self-observation rooted in the oldest form of meditation. Based on the ancient philosophy, our earliest traumatic memories begin in childhood and create a "scar or ridge" in the brain called *Sankhara*, in Pali language, or *Samskara*, in Sanskrit. The theory is that if this scar or trauma goes untreated, we move through life triggering the unhealed wounds and traumas. With each struggle, the scar becomes deeper and our suffering continues. Scientifically, these are the neural pathways of our brain that are triggered. The neural pathways connect one part of the nervous system to another. The pathways become used in reaction to any trauma. With mindful observation and meditation, we can help change these pathways and create new ones. Once the new pathways are created, we can use them to redirect the thought process and introduce mindfulness. The discipline of meditation helps to train the brain to observe sensations which are triggered by thoughts and to learn to let them go.

Further, the technique trains us to learn to avoid attaching or repelling any thought that may come up and deepen the ridge. This comes from practice and observation of the thoughts. It is a scientific method of preventing the same neural pathways from being constantly triggered. When the pathways are triggered, the mind revisits the downward spiral of negativity. The trauma and negativity keep us stuck in unhealthy and unhelpful thinking patterns which in turn perpetuates our suffering.

Meditation and self-observation are the ultimate goals of an aspiring yogi: one who practices yoga. The yoga practice which involves asanas or postures is another limb of the yoga philosophy. A successful yoga practice incorporates the same principles of meditation. In Vipassana meditation, we observe the breath and body sensations. The same principles are in a physical practice where we stay tuned to the breathing and the body sensations during each pose. The postures help to bring the mind into the present moment where past and future do not exist. Once we connect to the breath and body, we can determine the reality of the present moment as opposed to being lost in thought. The yoga practice is a mental process and at the same time scientific.

Through practice, the body's energy is balanced with decreased tension in the muscles, compression of veins, arteries, lymph nodes and glands which help to restore the natural flow and optimal function.

Stress and perpetual thinking not only decrease mental focus and cognition but also result in more tension in the body. Our brain's default mode can be described as mind-wandering. For most of us, even when we're doing nothing, our brains are highly active. Work projects, to-do lists and worrying about finances may feel like the norm but can be quite taxing on the brain. A specific area of the brain called the *default network* manages all that mind-wandering, and it requires energy and resources that are also needed for memory and cognition. Over time, the more energy and resources that go to the default network, the fewer you have available for paying attention and remembering other things. Furthermore, tension in the body limits proper blood flow. When there is limited blood flow, problems will soon arise due to inflammation and lack of circulation. Inflammation which goes untreated may lead to other illnesses and diseases.

Notice your physical body when you go on vacation and how some pain subsides. The nervous system tends to be in restore and recharge mode, blood flows freely, and pain may decrease due to reduced inflammation. Usually, after several days, the gut and digestive systems function better as well since they are intricately connected to the brain.

The "gut instinct" that we are all born with is the gift of intuition. It is an ability that can be easily ignored with a mind that is perpetually thinking. Presence practice, which is the practice of being in the moment, helps us reconnect to our power of intuition. We learn to listen to the body to help guide us. Studies have shown that there are the same types of cells in the information processing part of the brain as there are in the heart. So, the power and wisdom of allowing the heart to lead is supported by scientific reasoning.

HOW TO START A MEDITATION PRACTICE

Start your day by getting out of bed and onto a meditation cushion. Take advantage of the slow, waking mind and a nervous system that is calm. Once you are on your cushion or chair, sit upright without leaning back so the physical body is in an aware and graceful position. Begin by focusing on the breath and sense all parts of the body. Sensing the body begins with noticing tension and tightness and improving awareness skills to notice sensations such as heat, cold, tingling or vibrations.

The habit of a morning meditation will help you start your day calm, clear and aware. Start with ten minutes and work your way up to 30 minutes, then to one hour. It is also good to end your day with meditation back on the cushion or chair as opposed to laying down. Meditation should be done with full attention. End your day with focus on the breath, clearing the mind and bringing attention back to the breath and back to the body. Again, begin with ten minutes and work your way up to 30 minutes.

Developing the practice of breath awareness and stillness helps reduce agitation, disturbances and anxiety. We can then accept that thoughts are just thoughts. These thoughts change and they come and go. We learn to avoid attaching or identifying with each one. We give the thought space, and we reduce our suffering. We find more moments of peace and balance. With awareness practice and equanimity, we learn to manage life's challenges with more agility and less resistance.

I personally prefer to begin my day with meditation and continue with a physical yoga practice. A beginner sequence is outlined at the end of the book. This simple routine will help you to start your day feeling calm mentally and energized physically.

5. Hatha Yoga
Physical Practice and Breathing Techniques

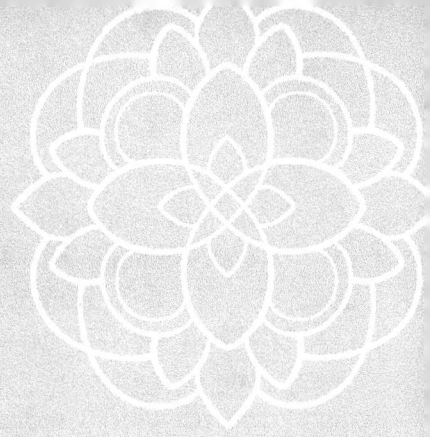

"Awareness is the Greatest Agent for Change."
~ Eckhart Tolle

Hatha Yoga is a branch of yoga that includes Asanas, which are physical postures along with Pranayams, which are breathing techniques. The Sanskrit translation for Hatha is *fierce and forceful*. For a nurturing practice, avoid forcing the body past its capability. Work the body with honest effort to find the strength and flexibility through a regular practice, always with the intent to avoid injury and self-harm.

Hatha, pronounced Hah-dha, was developed in India more than one-thousand years ago. The physical practice was intended not only to help alleviate pain in the body, but also to prepare the body for meditation in a seated position. It was acknowledged early on that most adults cannot comfortably sit on the floor in a cross-legged easy pose.

When we have overwhelming pain in the body, it is challenging to care for the pain in others. We get caught up in our pain-body both mentally and physically and therefore cannot be of service to others. Some studies have shown that inflammation in the body is closely related to inflammation in the mind. The inflammation in the mind can contribute to depression and ultimately to memory loss, dementia and Alzheimer's diseases.

The body cannot differentiate between various forms of stress. When we feel stress, it is translated in the body in the same way, whether the stress be emotional from relationships, a job, finances, or whether there is clear and present danger from a wild animal chasing you for its next meal. In times of stress and danger, the immune system shuts down, kidneys shut down, the breath becomes short, and the heart starts pumping harder and faster. This is beneficial for us to run away quickly and is a necessary adaptation for our survival. Yet sustained stress over time will break down the body, weaken the immune system and result in the body succumbing to disease.

Physical awareness gives us information on how the body is feeling and, in turn, we can determine what the body needs and wants. Mental awareness helps us process information at a conscious level and replaces old patterns of reactivity and belief systems. When we are completely aware in the present moment, we discover a space of no judgment or hatred. Judgment and hatred and other negative thinking come from subconscious and unconscious thought patterns and belief systems. We are not born with belief systems, so we can choose to change them as we start to wake up and become more conscious.

It is helpful to understand the three tiers of consciousness from a philosophical perspective. We are born conscious and slowly become aware of sensory perception and the thought process. As we move through life, we accumulate experiences that make impressions in our mind. As these impressions are made, we connect them to *good* and *bad* or positive and negative experiences. The good experiences, we try to recreate; the negative ones we tend to suppress. The suppression of our experiences creates samskaras, or in scientific terms, neural pathways. To clarify, the three tiers of consciousness can be compared to the following: at the unconscious level we have blinders on and cannot see, at the subconscious level we have tunnel vision and can only see what's in front of us, and through yoga and meditation we work on getting back to the conscious level, where we can see everything as it is and see it clearly.

HOW IS YOGA PRACTICE ACCESSIBLE TO ALL?

> It is through a yoga practice that we discover actual experiences of the mind and body, rather than adhering to a particular set of beliefs. "Therefore followers of all religions can benefit from the techniques. When practiced regularly, the methods of yoga lead unfailingly to deeper levels of spiritual awareness and perception." ~ *Paramahansa Yogananada*

For those of us looking to improve ourselves and find inner peace, whether through meditation or yoga practice, we need to begin with a commitment. Once you commit, it won't take long to discover and experience the immediate benefits. The practice of yoga reduces our physical pain, helps us clear the mind and calms the nervous system. With practice we create mental, emotional and physical space. In this space we connect to the deeper self. The deeper self sheds light back on love, humanity, compassion, peace and feeling connected with all living beings. In this deeper state we literally feel and understand that we are all part of One. We breathe the same air, and we breathe each other's breath. We are interconnected and interdependent of each other. We all suffer similar pains and joys and we know what it is to be human. We all essentially want the same things, including to love and to be loved. Yoga and meditation get us out of our heads and create some space. Space, stillness and silence are where we allow our brain cells to restore, to receive and to create again.

Some of us discover that we tend to spend much of our time in a state of fear, stress and even panic. In a state of fear, the brain does not function properly. Fear affects proper breathing. When the breath is inhibited and briefly stops, all functions of the body suffer, especially the brain. The brain needs most of the oxygen and water intake to run the entire body. The brain is the master gland of the body and signals all the other systems to function properly. Breathing brings oxygen to every cell of the body and our body needs oxygen to obtain energy to fuel all our living processes.

Our bodies are made up of 65 percent water and our brain is 75 percent water. Since our bodies are mostly water, even a small amount of dehydration can impair proper function. Considering these scientific facts helps us understand the effectiveness of deep breathing and proper hydration on the brain and body.

Meditation helps with focus and observation of the breath, while physical yoga helps with movement of blood and oxygen through the body. With this collaboration, the mind and body will function better to help us be happier and healthier beings. Without practice, we tend to forget the interconnectedness of these components of physiology.

Disturbance of the mind affects the body and a disturbance in the body affects the mind. With practice we acquire skills to improve the function of both the body and mind.

Pain

Pain sensations in the body help guide us through our practice. As new practitioners, some may identify each stretch and sensation as pain. A regular practice will help to identify which sensations are positive stretching sensations and which are just the body's way of communicating with us through pain.

A book that I recommend to students and practitioners is *The Gift of Pain* by Dr. Paul Brand and Phillip Yancy.[3] The book observes leprosy colonies worldwide. Leprosy is an infectious disease that affects the skin, mucous membranes and nervous system. The

---

3   Paul W. Brand and Philip Yancey, *The Gift of Pain: the Inspiring Story of a Surgeon Who Discovers Why We Hurt and What We Can Do about It* (Grand Rapids, Mich: Zondervan Publ., 1997))

attack on the nervous system causes lack of sensation and pain in the body. This lack of sensation allows a patient to quickly go from a small cut at the bottom of the foot that goes unnoticed to a severe infection which can lead to amputation. Understanding the disease magnifies the importance of pain sensations. When the pain is felt, understood and respected, the body has a chance to heal. When we feel pain, we are notified that something is wrong and to tend to this pain. The pain sensations help to protect the body from further damage. Pain is our warning system for self-preservation and ultimately survival.

With sensitivity and awareness during a physical yoga practice, the sensation of pain tells us to back off. Once we get more comfortable with the poses, it's important to be able to breathe throughout the pose. If the breath becomes labored, it is an indicator to back off. The connection to the breath serves as both a meditation and as a signpost to guide you during practice.

There are some postures with intentional compressions that may alter the breath, but this is a rarity as opposed to a norm. With good instruction, you will know when the altered breath becomes necessary.

Ahimsa is a Sanskrit word in yoga philosophy which means non-violence. One can observe it during practice by not inflicting pain or harm while trying to improve the body.

Pain needs to be respected and not ignored. A fundamental purpose of yoga is to connect body and mind, not to ignore the body for the benefit of the mind's egoic tendencies. So let the pain be your guide.

BREATHING TECHNIQUES

There are three breathing techniques highlighted below that can be practiced often. It is important with any and all breathing techniques not to force through any discomfort. For example, if you are a little congested due to allergies or a cold and having trouble breathing, you may consider skipping breathing exercises until the congestion has passed. If you notice that at any time during a breathing exercise it is difficult to find your breath, it's an indicator to stop the exercise and breathe normally until the discomfort passes.

Pranayama Deep Breathing

The sequence at the end of the book incorporates Pranayama deep breathing at the start. This technique helps build lung capacity by strengthening the diaphragm muscle. This method calms the nervous system and brings full attention to the breath. This can be practiced in a seated position or standing position. The movement of the arms helps facilitate the release of tension that builds up in the neck and upper back muscles. Many of us hold tension in this area as well as shorten our breath during high stress times. This is a great technique to either begin a sequence or for a quick break in your office chair. The steps are outlined in Chapter 12.

Kapalabhati Breathing

This breathing technique is also referred to as the *breath of fire*. With abdominal contractions, a bellows fan is mimicked, forcing air outward through pumping action. In the sequence outlined in Chapter 12, we end the series with quick exhale breaths to help release any free radicals that reside in the lung's lower regions. It helps build abdominal strength and coordination along with mental clarity and energy.

Alternate Nostril Breathing: Nadi Sodhana

This breathing technique results in mental clarity and promotes an even and smooth breathing pattern. I recommend practicing this method either at the start or end of a sequence or completely on its own. It's also very helpful to begin a seated meditation practice with this technique. Refer to Chapter 12 for step-by-step instruction.

6. Classical Yoga
The Philosophy

"Being spiritual has nothing to do with what you believe
and everything to do with your state of consciousness."
~ *Eckhart Tolle*

The philosophy of yoga guides us to live a more conscious life rather than subscribing to a particular belief system. This element differentiates yoga philosophy from a religion. The yoga philosophy guides us to operate from a conscious level. Classical yoga is a system of spiritual knowledge through scriptures with the most notable, Patanjali's Yoga Sutras. The sutras highlight the yoga philosophy with the *Eight Limbs of Yoga.*

The eight limbs are steps designed in a particular order to train us for the more challenging levels. It guides us to begin with accepting responsibility for our actions, continues with methods to help clear the mind and finally prepares us to live in a state of connection and bliss.

The Eight Limbs of Yoga are *Yama, Niyama, Asana, Pranayama, Pratyahara, Dharana, Dhyana*, and *Samadhi*.

The first limb, *Yama,* is about our attitude towards our environment — being of service to others, treating all our surroundings with respect, love and compassion.

The second limb, *Niyama,* is about our attitude towards ourselves. This includes treating ourselves with respect, love and compassion and taking care of our own physical, mental and emotional well-being.

The third limb is *Asana,* which is the physical practice of conditioning the body. It highlights respecting the body by taking care of our flexibility, strength and overall physical balance.

The fourth limb is *Pranayama,* which is restraint or expansion of the breath. It involves learning to observe, respect and understand the connection of the breath with the body and the mind.

The fifth limb is *Pratyahara,* which translates to sense withdrawal. The withdrawal of the sense is a mental practice to not react to stimuli from our senses. This practice is in preparation for meditation and settling the mind.

The sixth limb is *Dharana,* which is concentration. Learning to concentrate is even more imperative in our highly distracting world.

The seventh limb is *Dhyana,* which is meditation. The act of meditating brings mental and physical benefits of calming the nervous system, lowering blood pressure and working towards a clearer and stronger mind.

The eighth limb is *Samadhi,* which is the complete integration of all limbs of philosophy. Samadhi is the final step to becoming the most connected, self-realized, and self-aware. Samadhi is mastery of the mind.

Upon closer review of the *Eight Limbs of Yoga,* it makes sense why some people equate yoga with life. Following the guidelines can be a lifestyle, a choice for service to others and to ourselves which enables each one of us to live the best quality of life.

Classical yoga in India incorporated asanas, which specifically translate into seated positions. Before Hatha Yoga, meditation was considered the only form of yoga. The earliest yoga pose is the seated cross-legged pose. Variations evolved, such as the lotus pose which is the quintessential seated pose. Thousands of years later, classic yoga postures developed beyond seated postures.

Yoga philosophy is a way of life. It sets foundational practices to lead us towards more awareness and consciousness. The philosophy supports us to be more connected with ourselves, with others and within our environment. These "limbs" help set a path for less suffering. Following the philosophy, we discover ourselves at the deepest level. When we function from a place of connection, we can better serve ourselves, each other, Mother Earth, and all living beings. The connected space is consciousness.

7. Modern Yoga
What is it and How was it Influenced?

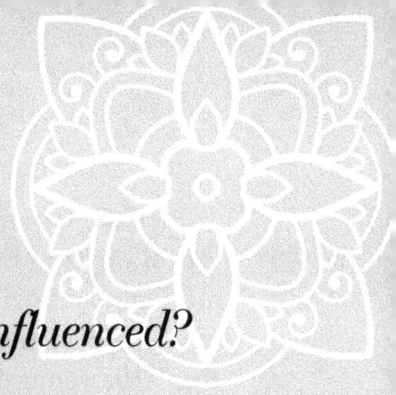

Modern yoga is generally considered the current day Vinyasa Style. Vinyasa is also known as *flow yoga* which refers to the movement of body with the breath. Vinyasa stems from the Krishnamacharya lineage. Tirumalai Krishnamacharya was a twentieth century Indian teacher who was referred to as "The Father of Modern Yoga." He was an influential yoga teacher who helped foster Pattabhi Jois and Ashtanga yoga, B.K.S. Iyengar and Indra Devi.

Physical or Hatha Yoga emerged around 5,000 years after the introduction of meditation and yoga philosophy. Hatha Yoga further developed through the Dutch colonization of India (from 1605-1825) which influenced gymnastics and calisthenics techniques.

The Dutch had economic and social influences through the establishment of the Dutch West and East India Trading Company. The Dutch introduced not only economic and social changes in India but also a physical culture through gymnastics and calisthenics. About 25 years after the Dutch influence, the British colonization of India took place from 1858-1947. The British also had direct influence over the modern-day yoga style. The physical training of the British soldiers, specifically push-ups, helped develop their muscular physique, so the wiry-bodied yogis learned to incorporate more workouts that the British soldiers were performing. The British introduction of push-ups were incorporated into the modern-day yoga sequence known as Sun Salutations. The Sun Salutations are a series of postures that incorporate push-ups and stretching to build upper body strength and flexibility.

In 1923, Paramahansa Yogananda, not only founded the College of Physical Education in Calcutta but later became one of the most famous Yogis who ventured to the United States. Yogananda wrote one of the most prominent books, "Autobiography of a Yogi". His younger brother, Bishnu Charan Ghosh was an Indian bodybuilder and Hatha Yogi who developed the Ghosh lineage which later contributed to the Original Hot Yoga.[4]

The integrity of yoga is based in ancient Indian philosophy, but upon delving deeper, the more popular styles were influenced by the events transpiring within India's political system and more specifically during the colonization periods.

Many of the physical yoga sequences incorporate breaks or Savasanas, which help the postures in their effectiveness. Savasana is a meditative resting posture lying on the back which offers a short break within or at the end of a sequence. The more modern styles were inspired by calisthenics through British influence. The Vinyasa style, or connecting postures with the breath, is a modern label on how to gracefully move through the postures and transitions. The Ghosh lineage weaves numerous breaks between the postures, especially during the floor sequences. This break allows for the circulatory system to assist in recovery following the compression effects of the poses.

To simplify the workings of a physical yoga practice, the basics are within a seated meditation approach. Physical yoga incorporates postures while maintaining the awareness of the breath. The movements are slow and mindful. Breath observation during physical practice assists in calming the body and mind through the nervous system while challenging the body to improve strength and stamina performing each pose. The physical yoga practice emulates meditation practice with breath observation and body sensations.

---

4   Mark Singleton, *Yoga Body the Origins of Modern Posture Practice.* (Oxford: Oxford University Press, 2010)

Normal breathing and proper oxygenation help the body increase stamina, allowing for longer sustained practices. Physical yoga practice helps us build strength, create flexibility and, most importantly, connect to the body.

In some yoga venues, the direction of yoga is now in the speed of the movement and the volume of the music. Ultimately, yoga practice and meditation practice should be done in silence. The silence and space are needed to observe the breath, to slow the thoughts (without introducing new ones) and to rid the body of tension.

Music has an emotional and sometimes a nostalgic effect. The nostalgia takes our mind into a different moment, extracting us from the present moment. This can trigger the subconscious mind that may lead into a string of other thoughts. The goal of yoga practice is to train the mind to be present, aware and undistracted. It is important to avoid altering the emotional state with more distractions or in some cases, memories.

The practice of presence is where we want to be. On many occasions, music will bring us to a pleasant thought and experience but to train the brain to be present in the moment, it is important to avoid thoughts that introduce attachments to the past. These are results of an untrained mind. The thoughts contribute to our desires, and this further contributes to the constant fluctuations of the mind. These fluctuations ultimately bring suffering, misery and sadness that take us out of the present moment.

Instructors and guides who teach to the public would benefit from avoiding scents and fragrances that both distract the mind and may be harmful to some practitioners. The fragrances may include essential oils, incense and scented candles. Most often, we are not made aware of allergies or illnesses students may have, whether they be physical or emotional.

Our senses contribute to subliminal thoughts and emotions. These thoughts are sometimes associated with samskaras, or neural pathways, that have been created from past experiences. These past experiences can contribute to our lack of presence at any given moment. Therefore, in physical and meditation practice, it is important to eliminate all distractions and to create a quiet space.

Pandit Rajmani Tigunait discusses how Samskaras can affect us and our choices:

> Is a samskara something you must live with because it is your destiny? Or is it like an old glove that you can avoid putting on?

> It depends on you. If you make the best use of all the potential you have as a human being, you avoid the effects of your samskaras. But if you are a fatalist, having no confidence in self-effort, then you will remain a victim of your samskaras. Let me explain.

> Samskaras are the subtle impressions of our past actions. As long as we are alive, we continuously perform actions, but not all of them contribute to the formation of samskaras. Actions that we perform with full awareness are the ones that make the greatest impression on our mind. In other words, it is the intention behind the action that gives power to that action. This process is beautifully explained by the literal meaning of the word "samskara." The prefix sam means well planned, well thought out, and kara means "the action under-taken." Thus, "samskara" means "the impression of, the impact of, the action we perform with full awareness of its goals." When we perform such an action, a subtle impression is deposited in our mindfield. Each time the action is repeated, the impression becomes stronger. This is how a habit is formed. The stronger the habit, the less mastery we have over our mind when we try to execute an action that is contrary to our habit patterns. We all have seen how our habit patterns subtly yet powerfully motivate our thoughts, speech, and actions.

8. Yoga Today
The Direction of Yoga and Meditation

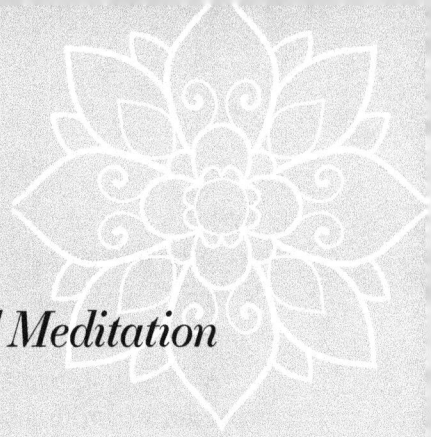

Many of today's yoga classes resemble aerobics and dance classes. The essential component of yoga as meditation and connection is watered-down or lost. The downside of our fast-moving world, and our bombardment of news and information, has created hyperactive minds that are agitated and in need of constant distractions. The discipline of sustained mental focus during practice is slowly fading.

The main component of yoga is about mastery of the mind which starts with quieting the mind. It has become a trend to not only have music in yoga classes but in some cases, loud electronic dance music. We all enjoy music, yet to experience an effective yoga practice, silence is necessary. It is this silence that most people resist settling into comfortably. If a studio or teacher is liked because of their playlist, that is not usually an indicator of a good studio or instructor. Teachers and fitness professionals love to be complimented on their playlists, but this would be more appropriate in a dance studio as opposed to a yoga studio.

DISTRACTIONS

The present day environment is filled with numerous distractions. It feels as if the latest fast editing style in films and television programs resembles our daily lives. The influx of information, the progression of technology and the constant need for new distractions has contributed to unsettled minds and overactive nervous systems. We are bombarded with news and information that is usually irrelevant to our individual daily lives and we are surrounded with new trends that are ultimately driven in pursuit of financial profit.

Access to information and exposure to new experiences has increased with the progress of technology. We are bombarded with advertising in all forms. Many people are manipulated by ads for the latest high-priced handbag (that a celebrity carries) and believe it to be exactly what is needed to make them feel important. These are all distractions — ways for us to live through a fantasy or belief system and reject our own reality.

If you are one who reflects and seeks a life of growth and wisdom, the realization may arise that much of your idea of life is built on fantasy. The disappointment of reality not matching the fantasy is what brings much of the conflict within. The path of yoga helps resolve these conflicts.

Many young children are exposed to stories that help form fantasies through books and movies. These fantasies are further sold to us through media and advertising. Yet it is important to take responsibility for our own thought process. We can choose to believe these stories or instead choose to use our independent minds to decide our path. Sooner rather than later, AI, or artificial intelligence, may possibly take over our thought process. So, you can make the decision now to maintain your individuality and independence or you can choose to be controlled by outside influences.

Yoga helps us to see things how they really are, to see reality as it is and to sit with it. We learn to appreciate our bodies, our breath and the present moment. This is how peace is introduced back into our lives. This is what yoga is about and what meditation is about. It takes us out of our hypnotized state and brings us back to the present moment. We distract ourselves and attach meaning to ideas to get out of feeling what is happening right now.

A strong yoga and meditation practice will help us have fewer attachments to stories and belief systems along with fewer attachments to the past and future. Life is happening now, and it is not happening when you get the new job, new house, new relationship, or the perfect body. We are constantly distracting ourselves from the present moment due to conditioning and belief systems that do not serve us or even pertain to us.

Currently, the principles of yoga are being ignored and worse, even unknown. Whether we live now or lived thousands of years ago when yoga began, we need the foundations of practice, discipline, and awareness in daily life.

If you have had the opportunity to take horseback riding lessons, you may be familiar with how to instruct the horse. If you ask the horse to gallop or trot, there are verbal sounds or cues given to the horse. The cue is not given once, but it is given repeatedly to maintain the desired outcome. This is the same with our human minds. We need to discipline the mind constantly to keep the circuitry and the desired outcome consistent. This is why meditation is meant to be a daily practice. We need to clear the mind because every event and experience can be a distraction, especially for an untrained mind.

We worry, stress and create a lot of unneeded anxiety because we think we can control outcomes with our thoughts. We make ourselves miserable by giving in to distractions in our minds just because we have a hard time sitting with the myriad of emotions that may come up. Each experience in our lives has layers of emotions. As we experience life, if we are tuned into our emotions and thought processes, we see that events that should bring us happiness sometimes bring up a lot of sadness as well. As the restless beings that we are, we may finally reach a goal or a desired outcome and yet we almost immediately forget and rush to find something new to distract ourselves with. Being is a state that most people have trouble with. Yoga helps us to do this. Not just through the physical practice, but especially through a disciplined practice of meditation.

Meditation helps bring us back to the present. Meditation helps us to learn to observe the distracted mind while physical yoga helps us to focus the mind on one pose and one breath at a time. The physical yoga practice helps us get to the sitting meditation practice which is more difficult to do. Sitting still is difficult and focusing on the breath for more than a minute is difficult. Anything difficult needs to be practiced with diligence and repetition.

In 2013, I held my first retreat in Santa Barbara. I attempted to hold my first guided meditation session with a group of students who had years of physical yoga experience. I made the mistake of giving limited verbal instruction. I introduced the few meditation guidelines and remained silent until the end. As I recall, the session was for about 15 or 20 minutes. Most of the students were not only frustrated but clearly did not enjoy the experience. Recalling the various complaints I received, I remember one student who was a notable film and television actress at the time. She was so frustrated by the experience that she could not stop complaining for what felt to be nearly an hour. It was interesting not only to witness the discomfort which results from sustained silence, but the results of creating a quiet space and witnessing the lack of discipline from a seasoned group of yoga practitioners! It was clear that a strong physical yoga practice had little to do with the discipline of a seated meditation practice. It proves that everything needs attention and practice, even sitting in silence and breathing. Hatha Yoga was designed to guide us more effortlessly towards the discipline of seated meditation, and this was a clear indicator that I had to incorporate more guided meditation classes in my program.

Distractions can come in many forms. They can come from constant noise, movement, visuals, stimulants, drama, people, experiences, and traveling. In other words, anything and everything can serve as a distraction. That's why even five minutes in the morning and five minutes in the evening can help us create a little bit of space. This space is needed from the incessant noise and distractions that keep us from experiencing the present moment as it is. In the present moment, most of us are lucky to have a roof over our heads, food and nourishment in our bodies and loved ones in our lives. Essentially, we do not *need* anything else.

Paramahansa Yogananda who wrote *Autobiography of a Yogi,* was one of several Indian yogis to introduce yoga philosophy and practice to the United States. Below is a quote that highlights the benefits of yoga practice and the connection to finding wisdom and fulfillment in life.

> It is not a pumping in from the outside that gives wisdom; it is the power and extent of your inner receptivity that determines how much you can attain of true knowledge, and how rapidly. You can quicken your evolution by awakening and increasing the receptive power of your brain cells.

> Most of us are accustomed to looking outside of ourselves for fulfillment. We are living in a world that conditions us to believe that outer attainments can give us what we want. Yet again and again our experiences show us that nothing external can completely fulfill the deep longing within for something more."[5]

---

5 Paramahansa Yogananda, *Autobiography of a Yogi* (S.l.: Ancient Wisdom Publication, 2019)

9. Our Compass
How to get Back on the Path

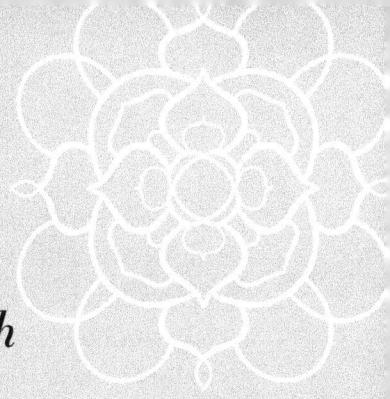

"Always say 'yes' to the present moment . . .
Surrender to what is. Say 'yes' to life —
and see how life starts suddenly to start working
for you rather than against you."

~Eckhart Tolle

What is the path? The path is to recognize our true, deeper and conscious self. To know that we are whole and to learn to trust our own internal guide. The path is where we can live a healthy, honest, balanced and fulfilled life. It takes dedication to oneself to build the discipline of self-awareness and self-reflection. Yoga philosophy guides us to act in a way that supports us and the people around us without causing injury or harm to any living being. This is the first step to creating a healthy internal and external environment.

Due to the progress in technology and available information, our world is changing at an increasingly fast pace. We can adapt by learning to grow with progress. The most important part for our evolution is to stay connected to our humanity and build strong emotional health within ourselves and especially in our kids.

The negative effects of technology can be witnessed at the emotional level with young kids, pre-teens, teenagers and adults. Technology is designed to be a benefit to everyday life, but all things have positive and negative results. Technology makes our lives easier in many ways yet contributes to our minds becoming lazier. The current debate over advertising algorithms geared towards young kids and teenagers is something we need to stay educated on. Technology designed to manipulate our emotions or habits is important to avoid. Many social media platforms are engineered to trigger us emotionally. That is what advertising goals are geared towards, to affect us at an emotional level so we act. Notice that most advertising reinforces that we need more "things" to be happy. The messaging is based on belief systems that are not only untrue but designed to make money for large companies.

Meditation and yoga will be more relevant in the coming years to counteract the negative impact that social media and technology can have. The warning signs of social media and technological manipulation include extreme cases that end in suicide and violence, especially among teens and young adults. The mental and emotional disorders that result can be avoided with more emotional connections and practices.

How we stay on the path demands awareness of oneself, awareness of our triggers and our thoughts about ourselves. It's important to differentiate what is one's own truth and what is just noise. Noise tends to trigger us, upset us, even make us temporarily happy. Yet when you know your truth, when you maintain connection to your deeper self, you build your own power and resilience to outside influences. This work on yourself will not only reinforce mental and emotional health but will lead you to a place of balance and calm. Yoga and meditation practice is a form of empowerment. We connect to our deeper self and no longer give our power away to other people. Giving our power away not only derails us from our path but depletes us mentally and emotionally.

Fear may come up often through our challenges. Although fear is an important survival mechanism, if unobserved, it can distract us from our path. Fear sometimes derails us and keeps us from moving towards our purpose or our deepest desires. Fears and doubts hinder us, even weaken us, and if gone unchecked may make us unhappy and ultimately depressed. If we allow ourselves to stay in a fear state, we become paralyzed mentally, emotionally and physically. In this state, we tend to restrict life from unfolding naturally. Consistent practice of meditation and yoga, self-refection and healthy living help us to settle into the now and stay on our path.

COMFORT IS DEATH

There are three words that made an impact on me the first time I had heard them. I have used these words in the past to help students through challenging yoga classes. These three words are *comfort is death*. The phrase was introduced to me over 20 years ago and is a constant reminder of growth and discipline. When students would first hear me use this phrase in class, they would think I was crazy, but soon came to understand what was meant at a philosophical level.

The Physical

The practice of yoga is not comfortable. The body struggles to regain strength and flexibility which it loses over time. From a novice point of view, the sensations are identified as pain. Once the sensations of stretching and strengthening are differentiated, then one can identify good pain from bad pain. The original Sanskrit term for physical yoga, Hatha Yoga, means fierce and forceful. This is important to get the body back in working order. The intensity of a practice will strengthen muscles and promote circulation which improves proper functioning and optimal energy back to the body.

Although intensity is needed for building strength in the muscles, it does not mean that every practice must be forceful. Each practice is based on the level of energy you may have on any given day. Some days you may need to not hold postures as long and some days you may need to hold stretches a little longer.

With more practice and honest effort, you will learn to tune into the body's needs. The balance of strength and flexibility will ultimately bring the body back to proper functioning.

The Mental

From a philosophical and mental perspective, we experience events in our lives where we may feel we are not challenged. We tend to fall asleep, hypothetically. Prolonged complacency may lead to unhappiness. Studies have shown that people who seek to learn and grow not only help the cognitive brain but also tend to suffer less with depressive disorders. The cognitive mind is the design of the brain's function. Cognition is the mental action or process of acquiring knowledge and understanding through thought, experience and the senses.

To compare our yoga practice to life, notice that a healthy practice changes and evolves as well. Age happens, injuries happen, and so does illness but we modify the poses to accommodate the body when needed. For many of us, to do something less, when necessary, is just as important as knowing when to continue to push for more. In yoga practice, our minds should not dictate the body but collaborate with the body.

A strong yoga practice is achieved by listening to the body through the senses and working with what is happening on each given day. Please don't make the common mistake of working with the body on how it was a year ago or last week or how you want it to respond next week. A large part of meditation and yoga philosophy is to accept things as they really are and observe without judgment. Judgments are mind-made concepts that do not serve us in our yoga practice.

For example, if you are recovering from an injury, approach the pose slowly and hold the pose wherever possible with focus on the breath. Stillness, breath, and observation are all very uncomfortable for most of us yet encapsulate the necessary ingredient of yoga and meditation.

Yoga is a personal practice. Yoga was originally designed to be practiced one on one: teacher and student. The group class was a way to reach more people efficiently in one session. Both yoga and meditation practice can be done in groups and in solitude. Even if you are one who enjoys group classes, try to balance it out by doing a personal and or private practice at least once a week. You will discover different levels of focus, concentration and even energy.

The path of meditation and yoga leads us to the deeper or higher self. The self that has no name, no past and no future but is the witnessing presence in the background. When we quiet the mind, we can listen to our heart and tune into the universe's guidance. We are intuitive beings, able to feel what is right for us as long as we can quiet the noise and go inside. Our soul is unchanging, steady, calm, connected and loving. We have an internal compass yet, with too much thinking, doubting, worrying and distractions, we lose focus. Our practice can help us tap into our heart, our soul and our intuition. Our soul is not attached to ego, how we look, where we go and what we own. Meditation helps quiet the distracted mind and reconnect us to where we belong.

PRACTICE SILENCE

The practice of sitting in silence is not only necessary but very therapeutic. How often do you sit and just observe your breath? The quieter we become, the louder the thoughts become. The act of meditation not only helps acknowledge the constant brain activity, but it helps you to gauge where you are daily.

You may ask, "What are the health benefits for sitting in silence and observing the breath?" It helps to bring your heart rate down, lower blood pressure, and strengthen the immune system. Meditation and breath observation need to be done daily for the best results. The mind is an organ yet needs to be worked like a muscle to maintain strength. Doing it just one time or one week will help you notice the benefits, but it is important to make it part of your daily life for long-term results.

Our environment with technology and social media is very noisy and can be extremely distracting. Distractions may be toxic and pave the way to disconnection and lethargy. When the mind is unfocused and filled with too much unnecessary thinking, the overall body energy decreases. Unfortunately, most thinking and mind-wandering usually leads to doubt, negativity and unhappiness. The habit of chronic thinking takes us out of the present moment. Just as we eat and sleep to maintain proper energy levels, yoga practice is a positive addition to maintaining higher levels of energy.

HABITS

Another benefit of meditation and awareness practice is noticing habits. An example of a good habit would be flossing our teeth after brushing. The habits I encourage you to notice are the negative ones. The most common negative habit is endless thinking patterns. These thinking patterns quite often turn into negative thinking patterns. They usually serve as a distraction to us. We can use a physical yoga practice to observe and temporarily stop these thinking patterns. At times, a yoga practice may seem extremely challenging mostly because of the distracted mind, so we practice reinforcing focus on breath and find that we can quiet the mind. Through the careful attention of our poses and our breath, we take the focus away from thinking and toward feeling. The physical practice lays the foundation for a meditation practice.

Many of us have reached pivotal moments in our lives where we notice that certain habits no longer serve us. Habits are usually automatic behaviors that we don't think about. Much of our practice helps us discover our negative and sometimes abusive habits and to learn to simply notice and ultimately let them go.

Whether you practice in a group or private setting, avoid making judgments and competing. Do your best to practice with integrity. Be honest with yourself about where your body is on any given day. Avoid allowing the ego (mind-made concepts about yourself) to guide your practice. Soon enough you'll notice that your practice will help guide you in your daily life.

When preparing for practice, please make sure your space is not cluttered and is clear of technological devices, mainly smart phones. It is important to learn to detach from everything to pay attention to your practice or meditation.

During my time as a studio owner, I would encounter a lot of resistance to students separating from their devices. We heavily enforced no devices to be taken into the yoga room. This was a courtesy to other students and especially to themselves. People get so attached to their smartphones that separating from them for an hour for class seemed like an impossible task.

Another very interesting thing that would happen is that students would get very attached to where they stood in class. Standing in the same space had become another habit that many could not part with. It's interesting how the habit of clinging and looking for comfort emerges repeatedly in various situations. I would even have students who would get into altercations about where they stood in class! I would regularly remind the students that no one owned real estate in the yoga room. This would give everyone a good laugh and highlight our automatic territorial tendencies. Habits create comfort zones for us both in positive and negative ways. Become aware of the unnecessary ones and even practice in different spots to avoid habitual tendencies.

YOGA AND DEPRESSION

One of the most noticeable results of yoga practice is increased energy and an overall sense of well-being. Much of this is due to the effectiveness of yoga on stress levels. As the stress levels decrease, the hormone levels become more balanced. Once hormone levels are more balanced, mood swings and irritability decrease. Much of our stress pushes us to resort to unhealthy activities. Some may turn to sugar, alcohol or drugs, which only result in imbalance and continued hormonal fluctuations and suffering.

All forms of physical activity help with balancing hormone levels, but with most sequences of yoga postures, poses will specifically compress and release areas of the body where hormone glands reside. The endocrine system is the chemical messenger system in the body. The endocrine glands located in the throat consist of the thyroid and parathyroid glands. The glands positioned in the skull are the pineal and pituitary glands. The glands located directly above the kidneys are the adrenal glands, and located deep in the abdominal cavity are the pancreas and the ovaries/testes.

Once the locations of the glands in our physical body are identified, the benefits of the poses tend to make sense. Yoga poses are a series of compressions. These compressions, with the combination of release and rest, allow for an increased flow of oxygen-rich blood to reach these specific areas.

As an example, backbends are one of the golden postures of any sequence. The backbend stretches the front side of the body from the throat all the way down through the abdomen and the front of the thighs. The opposite side of the body the posterior, benefits from a thorough compression. Stretch is created in the anterior, or front side of the body, and compression is created in the posterior, or back side of the body. A break or Savasana is highly recommended after a deep backbend to allow for the balance of the blood flow and to bring the spine back to a resting and neutral position.

This hormone balancing contributes to the overall positive sensations in the body and noticeably decreases the mental/emotional effects of depression.

Another major side effect of depression is low energy. With a consistent practice, energy levels increase. Unlike other forms of physical activity, yoga increases the body's energy levels by releasing tension and increasing blood flow. Tension can be compared to a dam within the physical body. Where there is a dam, the flow of blood and energy is hindered. Yoga postures essentially release the tension by lifting the dam to allow for the flow of oxygenated and nutrient-rich blood.

Learn to practice silence through meditation and yoga. Begin to notice habits and learn to change the mental patterns that keep you in a state of suffering. The path is clearer when you create the space to feel, reflect and improve your physical, mental and emotional state.

10. Self-Compassion
A True Art in Self Care

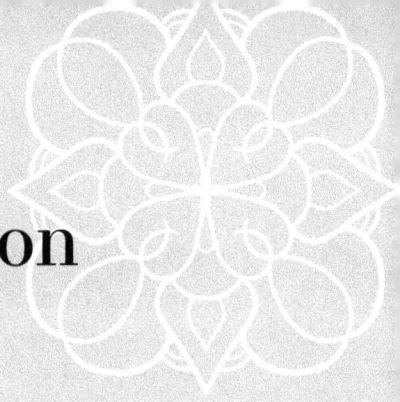

We are perfect in our being. Our being is our deepest self, the unchanging self, consciousness. As we evolve, we learn to examine our behaviors and belief systems. This self-reflection is often the root of our unconsciousness and suffering. The journey of self-reflection and self-observation, however, is best served by including self-compassion. Self-compassion involves learning to love ourselves, forgive ourselves, be kind to ourselves, and to ultimately stop the self-judgement and abuse that becomes part of our negative self-talk. Self-compassion is key to making our life journey a successful one.

Let's review the meaning of self-compassion before examining this subject a little more deeply. Compassion literally means *"to suffer together."* Among emotion researchers, it is defined as the feeling that arises when you are confronted with another's suffering and feel motivated to relieve that pain. Compassion is not the same as empathy. Although these two concepts are related, empathy is the ability to understand and share the feelings of another and take their perspective.

Having compassion for self is the same as having compassion for others. When we are suffering, we feel it, and are motivated to end the anguish for ourselves. To have compassion for others, first you must notice they are hurting, then you feel moved by their anguish and finally, the heart responds to their pain. You feel warmth and caring and the desire to help end the suffering for that person in some way.

Having compassion also means you offer understanding and kindness to others when they fail or make mistakes rather than judging them harshly. Finally, when you feel compassion for another rather than pity, it means you realize that suffering, failure, and imperfection are part of the shared human experience.

Self-compassion involves compassion towards yourself when you have a difficult time, fail, or notice something you don't like about yourself. Instead of just ignoring your pain with a stiff-upper-lip mentality, stop to ask yourself, "This is really difficult right now, how can I comfort and care for myself in this moment?"

Self-compassion includes being warm and understanding toward ourselves.

We, as humans, cannot always be as we want to be or get exactly what we desire. When this reality is denied or fought against, suffering increases in the form of stress, frustration, and self-criticism. When this reality is accepted with sympathy and kindness, greater emotional balance is experienced.

Suffering and personal inadequacy are part of the shared human experience. We all go through similar challenges in our lives, and it is important not to identify too closely with our own particular difficulties. When this perspective is incorporated, the challenge is simply that — a challenge — not something that defines us. You become aware of it instead of being overtaken by it.

FORGIVENESS

Forgiving means letting go of the protective armor of blame and/or hatred that encases your heart. Forgiving also means never putting anyone — including yourself — out of your heart. Forgiveness is also the compassion that arises when we've brought full presence to the suffering of hurt and wounds. I personally like to think of forgiveness as "open-hearted acceptance." The process of forgiveness unfolds over time.

Keep in mind that forgiveness does not mean we deny or suppress our anger, fear, hurt or grief. It does not mean we are passive or excuse harmful behavior. What is true for me is that my path of forgiveness hasn't happened all on my own. It has taken time and has required support. In addition to therapy and close friends, two of the main support systems for me are yoga and meditation.

Forgiveness is a tough topic for many of us, especially when it comes to family, loved ones, and even work relationships. Human conflict is a common struggle. In the extremes, it takes people and countries to war. I believe war and violence are the downfalls of humanity, and as we take a look around, we see they are a large part of history around the world. If we allow our hearts to be open and feel consciousness and our one-ness, we can agree that war and violence are appalling. Sadly, however, most of us do not have the power to change this.

We do have power over our own actions, thoughts, and behaviors. We all can work on loving-kindness and loving-compassion to affect our immediate surroundings and ultimately allow for those actions to expand and unfold.

We can take a look at our families and relationships. Notice where they may seem to be in conflict and struggling. This may be an area of your life where you may want to dig a little deeper. Doing so takes self-reflection, self-compassion, and avoiding blame and judgement. When addressing our relationships with others, it is important to first resolve the conflict within ourselves, and ultimately come from a place of love. Sometimes coming from the place of love may require us to give a little or a lot of distance. Finding the path that can give you the most peace is what is most important.

The interesting thing about forgiveness is that it gives *you* the most peace rather than the person being forgiven. It's powerful and life changing. Sometimes we need to remind ourselves that we no longer have a grudge against someone. We are all humans deserving of love, yet people's actions and behaviors may cause us pain. We can separate the action from the person and wish them well, learn to let go, and ultimately take care of our own emotional and mental well-being. Keep in mind that forgiveness is a part of our overall well-being and optimal health.

11. Surrender
Acceptance and Letting Go

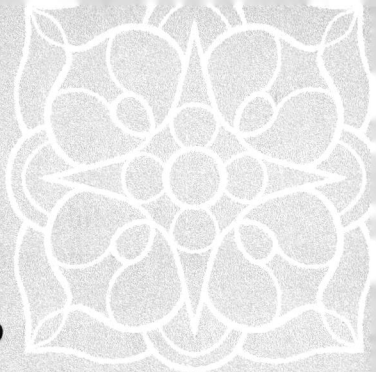

Practicing surrender is a recurrent theme within meditation and yoga. To transition from a place of resistance to a space of acceptance is the way to tune in to the present moment. Practice not labeling or judging the present moment and simply allowing it to be. This practice can be done at any moment in your day, especially when you notice struggle and dissatisfaction.

Meditation and yoga reinforce guiding the mind and body toward a calm and restorative mode for our nervous system. Through our practice, the feeling of home can be compared to a calm state of mind. Distractions, stories, negative feedback, and fear not only keep us in fight-or-flight mode, but they keep us from finding the home that exists within ourselves.

Much of our yoga, meditation, and life practice lies in the ability to surrender. Many of our struggles are rooted in resisting or attaching to events or situations. Through our practice of yoga and meditation, we learn to accept things as they are, and to ultimately surrender to what is.

It is important to remember that we are not surrendering to the event that causes our suffering. We must learn to surrender to the present moment, which is usually not the actual suffering itself. Most often, our present moment is exactly that. We may be working at our desks, cleaning, driving or any other activity. The suffering exists mostly in our minds. Each moment is a chance to tune into what is happening now.

A useful practice is to tune into the breath, sensations like sights and sounds, and our feelings at any given moment. Try asking yourself, "Where am I holding tension in my body at this moment in time?" The body and the breath are the most accessible ways to root us in the now. Much of our suffering is from *resistance* to the event causing the suffering rather than the event itself.

As we learn to move through life's challenges, it is helpful to remember that events and situations are in a constant state of change and movement. Allowing events to come and learning to let them go is a practice we master through our meditation sessions. The only difference is that the meditation practice is about allowing thoughts, rather than events, to come and go. This practice strengthens our resilience to life's struggles and stresses.

Much research has been done on scanning and observing the brain patterns of regular meditation practitioners. Mindfulness-based practices reduce activity in the amygdala, the area of the brain that governs stress response, fear and emotion. This reduction helps practitioners be less reactive to upsetting situations and to recover more quickly after a stressful event happens.

When we can avoid allowing our stressors to completely overwhelm us, we can stay rooted to our deeper self, our source, and allow the light of consciousness to shine through. When we are caught up in stories, patterns and behaviors, we tend to be lost and unaware of the real self. With closer examination, we may notice that our suffering lies in the stories we tell ourselves at that moment in time. The practice of meditation and yoga directly affect our daily lives by teaching us to let go of thoughts and recognize our levels of resistance.

Sometimes we feel overwhelmed by the idea that we need to "do" something about every situation or challenge. We feel we need to complete the story, fix the problem and end the suffering somehow. We often feel we need to rush through life. Once we have taken the action we may need to take as responsible human beings, it is important to step back and give it space. Recognize the challenge and give yourself time and space around this challenge. Not by obsessing, but by stepping back and allowing the natural process of the Universe to help you out. This may also be looked at as a way to surrender. You do your best, and then you step back and allow the process of life to happen.

Please note that this practice is effective for most of life's challenges, but not all. These guidelines are not for traumas, wars, and events that involve danger and death. Most of us are not dealing with life and death issues in our daily dilemmas. If we are, these challenges are best handled with a professional guide or therapist.

Therapy can also help us change our attachment and abandonment issues. Incorporating therapy sessions with mindfulness practices integrates the brain. Mindfulness and reflective work can aid in repairing samskaras, or physically change the neural pathways of the brain. With diligent practice, this helps us avoid *staying* in a suffering space.

One of the best pieces of advice I received from a close friend many years ago was that we often feel we need to do something, change something, or manipulate something to make it "work out" or to "fix it." The advice was, "Why don't you just do nothing?"

This gave me a moment of clarity and awareness. It really rang true for me because it gave me permission to step back and trust that the Universe will help sort it out. I don't necessarily need to take control every time.

One of my favorite sayings from Eckhart Tolle is, "Instead of asking, 'What do I want from life?', a more powerful question is, 'What does life want from me?'"

This, to me, is the start of *Surrender*, the embodiment of presence practice, and the way to Finding Home.

12. Your Way Home
Developing a Personal Practice

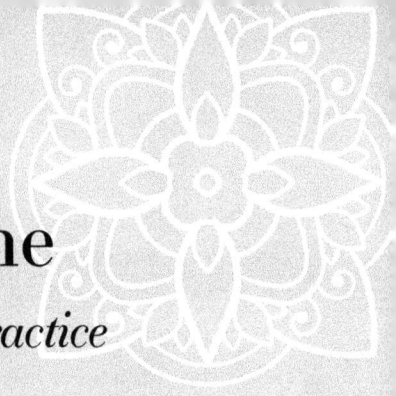

Yoga Practice facilitates movement of the body. Yoga strengthens and stretches all the muscles and therefore creates better mobility in all the joints. Please remember to notice and let go of ego and negative self-talk from your practice. One definition of *ego* is the part of the mind that mediates between the conscious and the unconscious and is responsible for a sense of personal identity.

Discomfort may be experienced during practice until the body's condition improves. Make sure to avoid pain sensations which resemble sharp and shooting pain. Pain is the messenger from the body to the mind, so build a healthy relationship by feeling and listening to the body throughout your practice.

For new practitioners, I recommend occasionally incorporating a practice in front of a mirror. The mirror can be used as a tool to help address proper alignment. Avoid criticism or judgment of the body and learn to love, appreciate and accept what you see. The body is an extraordinary vessel. Treat it well, take good care of it and it will be a much more comfortable space to inhabit.

Experiment with using props such as yoga blocks, yoga straps and, if needed, a yoga chair. Some practitioners who have a challenging time with balancing poses may consider using a chair until stability and strength are gained. Consider using these tools for assistance in executing the postures, but work with the intention of gaining full strength and mobility to someday practice without the use of them.

The body moves with greater ease when it is warm and generally in warmer climates. If desired, add a little heat and/or humidity for elevated levels of flexibility and sweating to help detoxify the body. Additional but not excessive heat will allow more stretch in the muscles and ultimately a better range of motion in the joints.

CREATING A SAFE SPACE FOR PRACTICE

To build an effective and strong practice, here are some basic guidelines:

1. The goal is to connect to Consciousness. The deeper self, the higher self, the witnessing presence.

2. Let go of the thinking mind. Yoga practice helps us practice *presence*. Being in the now.

3. Give it your honest effort. It is not easy. Growth happens with some discomfort. Hold each pose and focus on the breath.

4. Move slowly and mindfully. Enter and exit each pose slowly and with your breath. Avoid holding the breath.

5. Practice Ahimsa/Non-Violence. Avoid being aggressive with the body and acknowledge all sensations.

6. Learn to love yourself and your body with compassion and non-judgment

7. Avoid competing or comparing yourself to anyone else.

8. Practice with *mindfulness*. Be aware of your emotions and energy levels. They vary daily and can be affected by sleep, food, nourishment, weather and life events.

9. Hydrate properly and practice on an empty stomach.

10. Avoid stimulants such as caffeine and sugar before practice.

11. Avoid pain suppressants and vitamins before a practice.

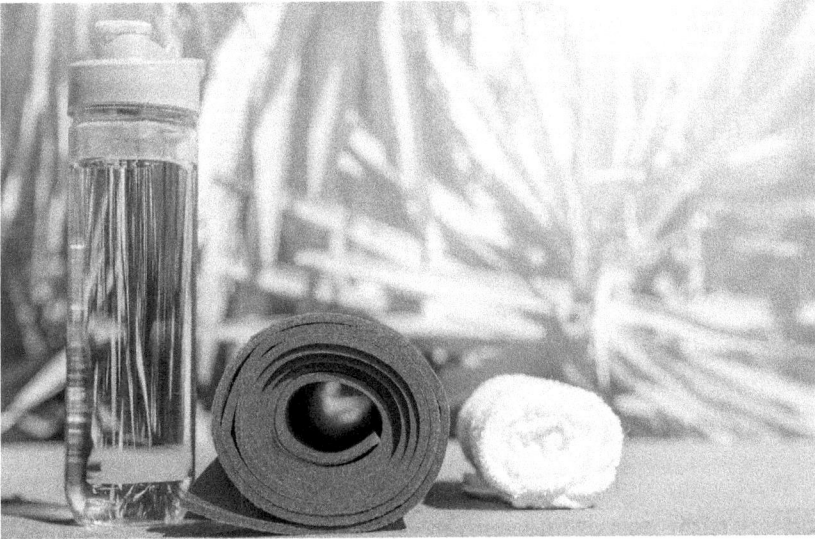

12. Avoid music for most of your practices. It is important to practice yoga and meditation in *silence.*

13. Find qualified instructors who communicate clearly and explain poses safely.

14. Avoid a search for a Guru. Find it in yourself. Instructors and guides are in service to students, not the other way around.

15. Advanced postures are appropriate with a dedicated and experienced practice. Avoid attempting advanced poses because of ego.

16. Practice *daily.* Unlike more common physical activities, yoga can be practiced every day.

17. Meditate every morning or daily. Even if it is only five minutes.

18. Use a mirror on occasion to check alignment and form.

19. Accept that each practice will be different, both physically and mentally.

20. Enjoy your practice! We tend to commit to things that we enjoy and make us feel good.

ALTERNATE NOSTRIL BREATHING

Below you will find the steps outlined for a very effective breathing exercise. As mentioned earlier in the book, this can be practiced on its own or at the start or end of a sequence.

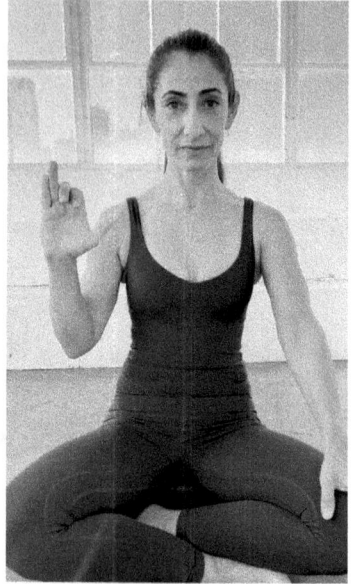

- Sit comfortably with a straight spine either in an easy pose or in a chair.

- With your right thumb, cover your right nostril and with a slight turn of the wrist, cover your left nostril with the pinky and ring finger.

- The index and middle finger can be folded inward or placed against the middle of the forehead between the eyebrows.

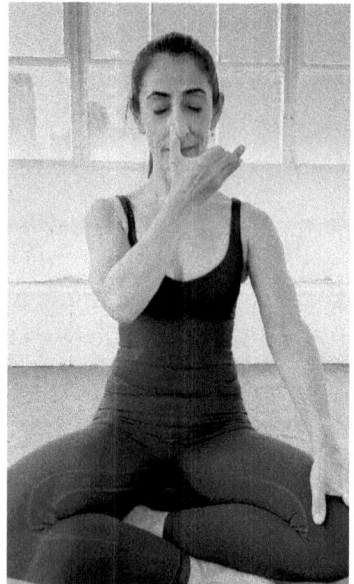

- The left hand can gently rest on your left thigh

- To begin, cover your right nostril and inhale fully through the left nostril up to a count of 4 or 5.

- Next, hold your breath and both nostrils briefly.

- Release the right nostril and exhale out for a count of 4 or 5. Stick with the same count each time.

- Follow this immediately by inhaling through the right nostril; hold briefly and exhale out through the left for a count of 4.

- This completes 1 cycle.

- Continue for 3 more cycles with eyes closed.

- Once the 4 cycles are complete, sit with your eyes closed and enjoy the sensation.

- When you are ready, slowly open your eyes and enjoy the renewed flow of energy.

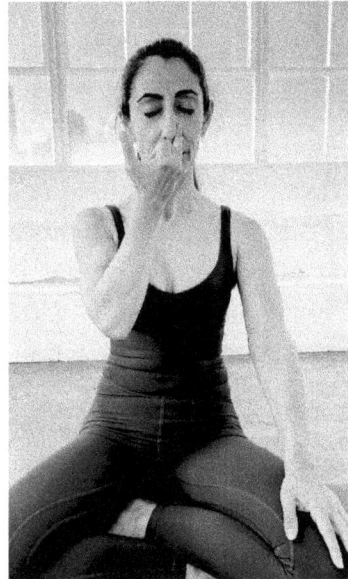

This breathing technique helps balance both the left and right hemispheres along with the breath. You will notice the flow of the breath becomes more even through both nostrils and the blood pressure is lowered. It is rare to not feel the benefits of this technique. Keep practicing and you will soon notice the difference.

SAMADI SEQUENCE LEVEL I

Please avoid using music. Get comfortable with silence and listen to your own breath.

For a longer, more effective practice, you may repeat these postures for a total of 2 rounds. Be sure to take 3-5 breaths between each pose.

1. Pranayama Deep Breathing

This breathing technique addresses the breathing apparatus which includes the lungs and diaphragm. Pranayama also helps the nervous system switch to the parasympathetic and calming mode. This way you can begin your discipline of focus and concentration. It also helps to alleviate tension in the most common areas of the body, the neck, shoulders and upper back.

- Begin standing with feet together, toes and heels touching. If balance is challenging, you may start with feet slightly apart.

- Interlace all 10 fingers underneath the chin while keeping the knuckles and chin in contact throughout the movement. Avoid having the fists against the throat.

- Looking forward, focus your eyes on one spot ahead and begin to inhale by the nose for 4–6 counts and lift the elbows up as high as possible. Inhaling slowly and deeply.

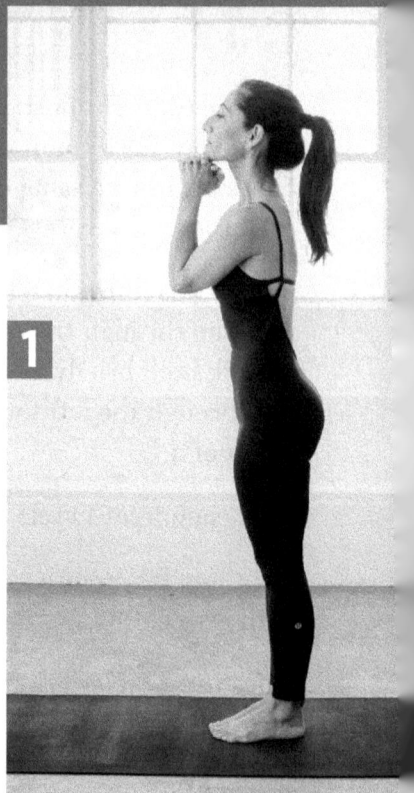

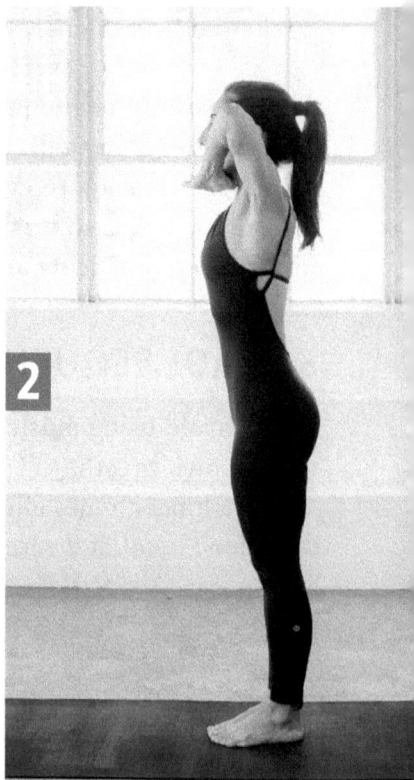

3

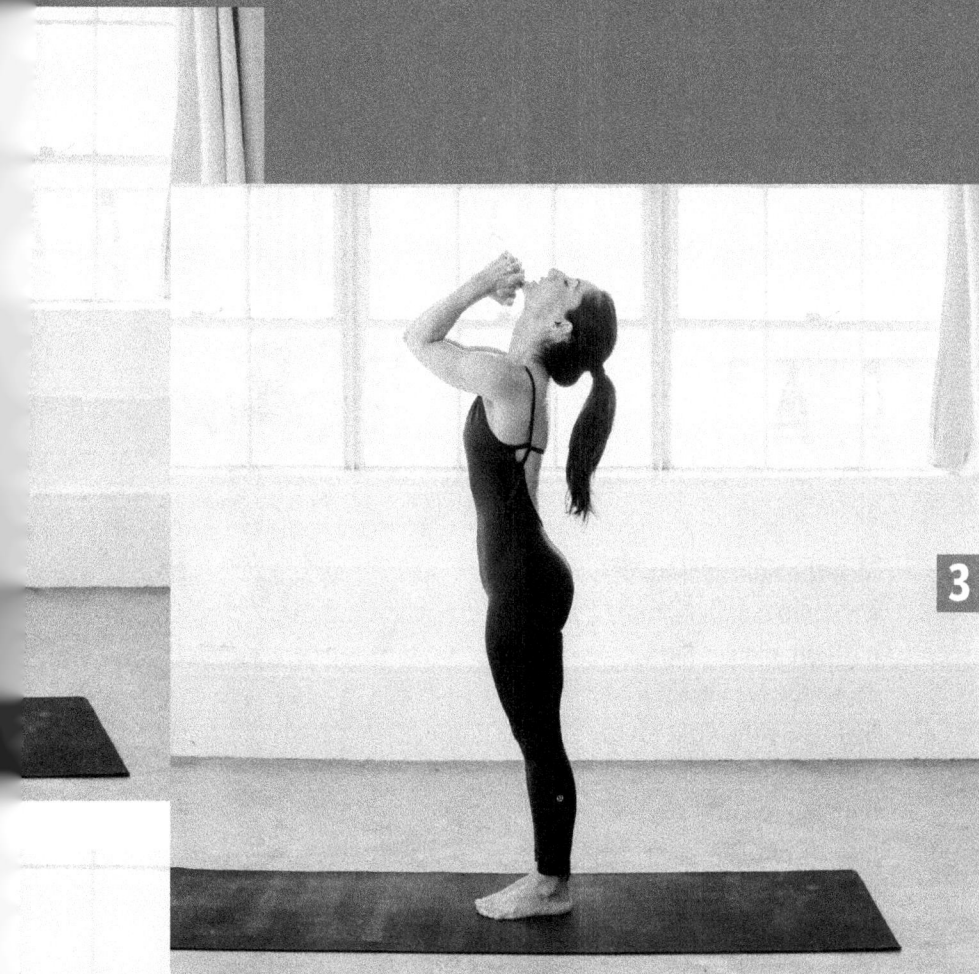

- As you exhale, open the mouth wide, exhale by the mouth and slowly push the head back as you bring the elbows to touch high in front and off the chest. If you experience discomfort in the neck, only tilt the head back to where it does not increase tension or pain.

Do 8–10 rounds.

2. Lunge

The lunge helps to stretch the hip flexors and demands the mental and physical discipline of balance.

- Begin standing with feet together and place hands on hips.

- Step the right foot forward into a high lunge position and get high up on the back toes. Make sure the right foot is directly ahead of the right hip and the knee directly over the right ankle joint.

- Keep the back leg straight with the back thigh muscle (quadriceps) contracted.

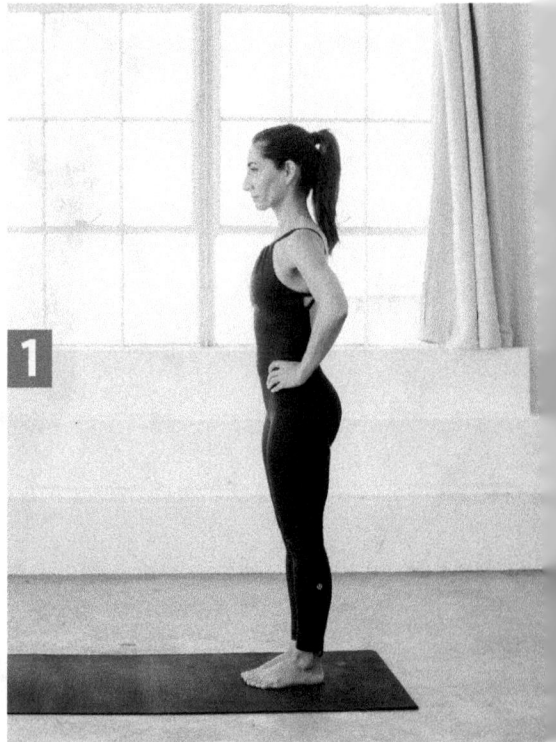

- (If there are any hip, knee or ankle injuries, you may take a smaller stance and keep the back foot flat on the floor.)

- Inhale the arms up overhead with the palms flat together (and thumbs crossed), and slowly move into a backbend. Hold for 3–5 breaths.

- Slowly move out of the backbend and step the left foot forward and the right foot back and repeat.

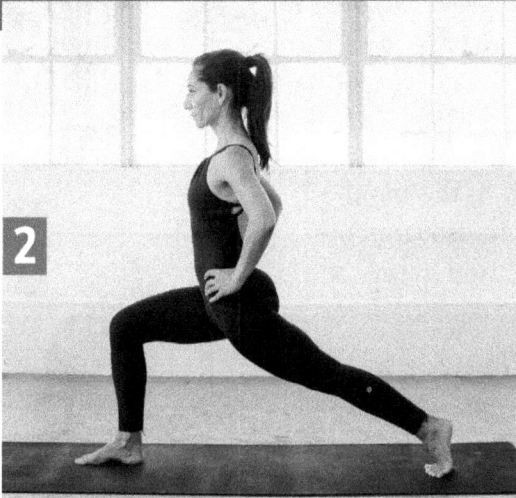

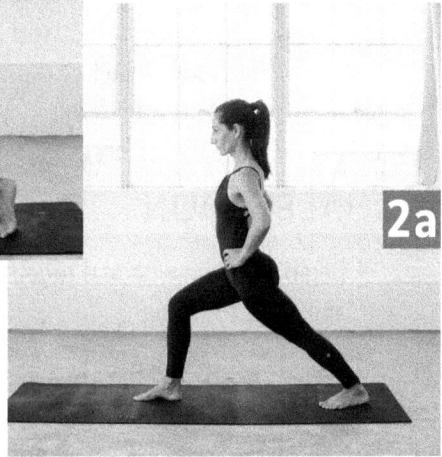

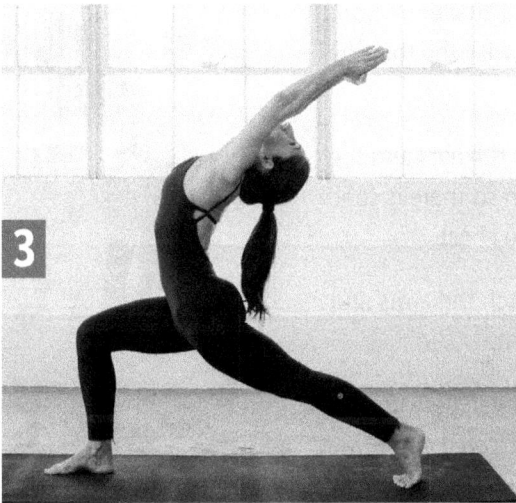

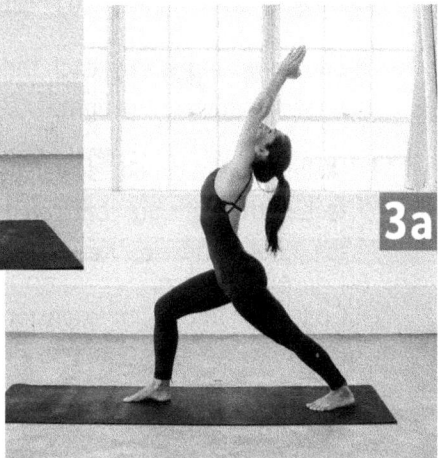

91

3. Half Moon Pose, Backbend and Hands-to-feet Pose

This pose helps mobility in the shoulders, spine and ribcage. It also stretches the upper body — upper and lower back — with an added compression to the kidneys and adrenals.

HALF MOON

- Begin standing with feet together and toes and heels touching.

- Inhale and extend the arms in straight position overhead. Interlace the fingers and release the index fingers while crossing the thumbs. For an additional challenge, you may keep the palms flat with the thumbs crossed or side-by-side.

- Keep the arms alongside the ears and the head in a neutral position so there is space between the chin and the chest.

- Stretch up and slowly reach the arms and fingertips toward the right.

- Make sure the weight is even between both feet, both thighs are contracted along with the gluteus muscles. Keep the abdominal muscles engaged.

- Go to your maximum extension and hold for 3–5 breaths.

Repeat by extending the body to the left.

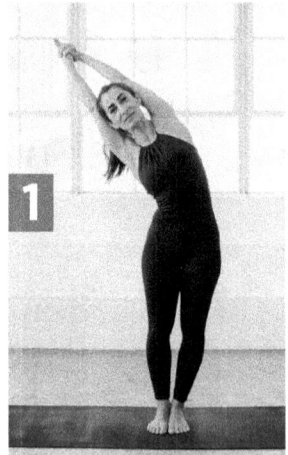

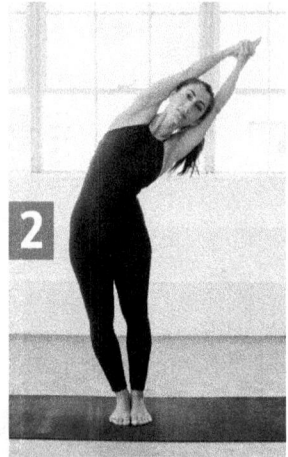

BACKBEND

- Keeping the arms extended up overhead, engage the gluteus muscles, lengthen up and keep the chest lifted and slowly move into a backbend. Bring the arms back as far as possible. Be sure to keep the chest lifted and push the hips forward as you bring the arms back. As long as there is no neck pain, you may let the head relax back, otherwise you may keep the head in line with the arms. Hold for 3–5 breaths.

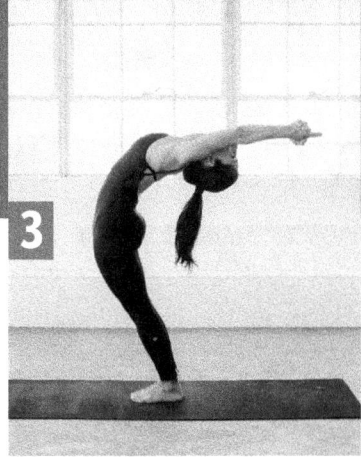

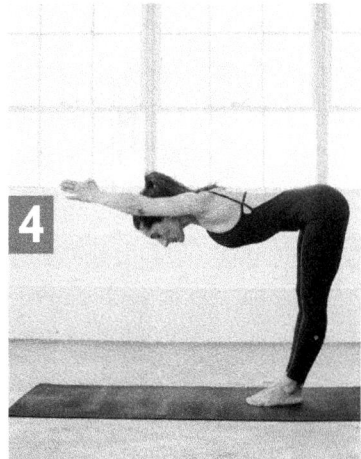

FORWARD BEND

- As long as there is no back pain or injury, try to move into the forward bend with straight arms, spine and legs. Otherwise move slowly, bending the knees and rounding the spine if needed. You may even walk the hands down the legs.

- Grab the heels (or as close to the heels as possible), stepping on all 5 fingertips of each hand. Ideally position the elbows behind the calves so that the upper body is in contact with the legs. Lift the hips and lengthen the spine straight down towards the floor. Hold for 3–5 breaths.

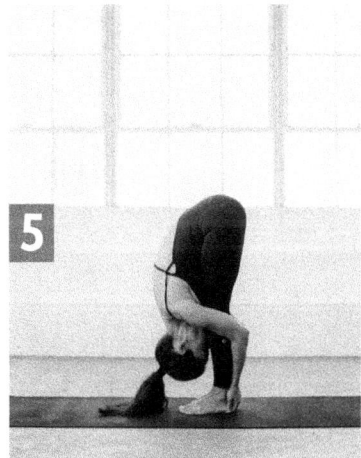

4. Chair Pose

This pose helps to strengthen the legs, release tension in the lower spine and increase the heart rate.

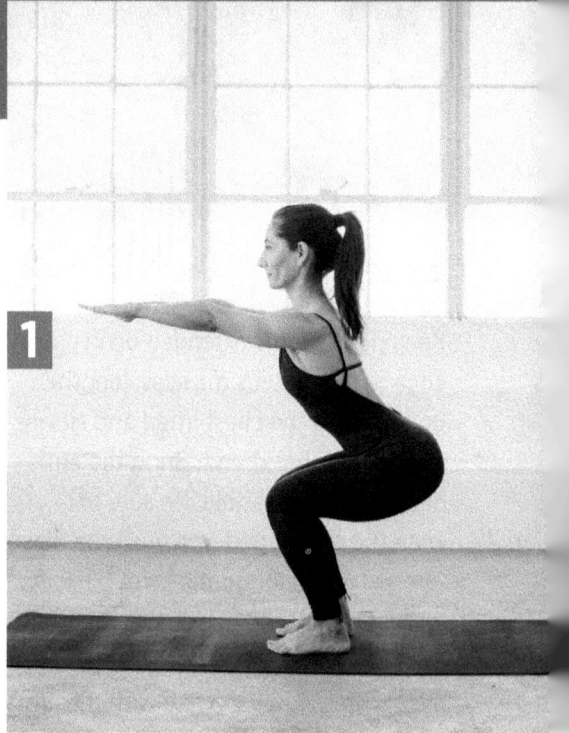

FIRST PART

- Step the feet about 6 inches or hip-width distance apart. Position the feet straight and parallel to each other.

- Inhale and lift the arms parallel to each other and parallel to the floor. Keep hands shoulder-width distance with the palms facing the floor and all fingers touching together.

- Exhale and simultaneously lower the hips as if sitting in a chair. Knees move forward directly over the toes and thighs parallel to the floor.

- To avoid strain to the knees, do not allow the hips to drop lower than the knees. This reduces contraction of the thigh muscles. Hold for 3–5 breaths.

SECOND PART

- Standing with feet hip-width distance, inhale and lift the heels up over the toes. Keep the heels in position and engage thighs, glutes and abdominal muscles for stability.

- Exhale and lower the hips down until thighs are parallel to the floor. Avoid lowering the hips below the knees. Stay up on the toes and hold for 3–5 breaths.

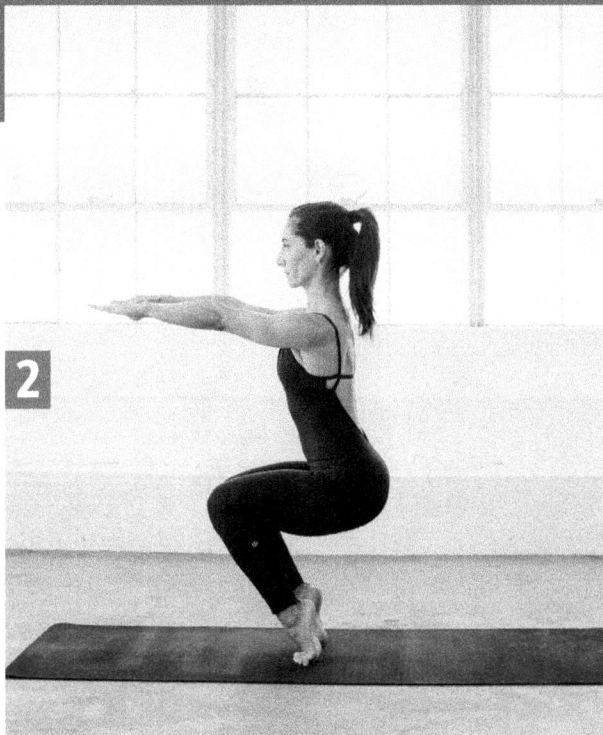

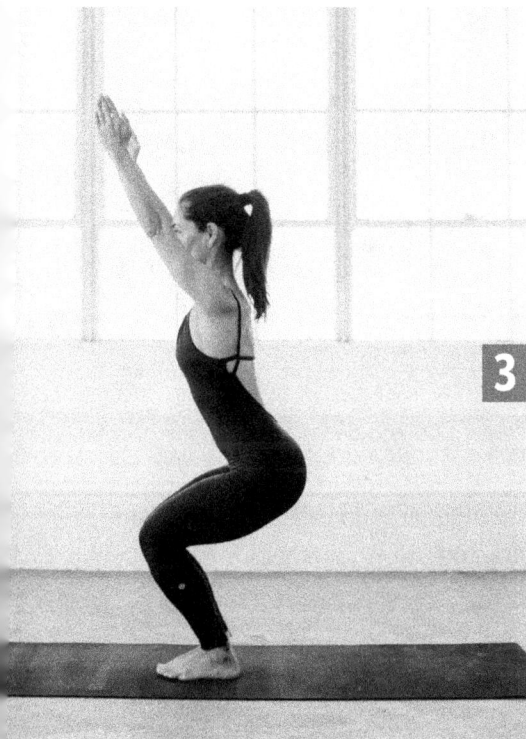

THIRD PART (CLASSIC CHAIR POSE)

- Stand with feet together. Inhale arms up and exhale to lower the hips down. Hold for 3-5 breaths.

Option: If there is knee pain or injury, keep the feet and knees slightly apart.

5. Eagle Pose

Eagle pose helps release tension in the upper back, improve the mobility in the shoulder and hip joints and promotes blood flow in the legs.

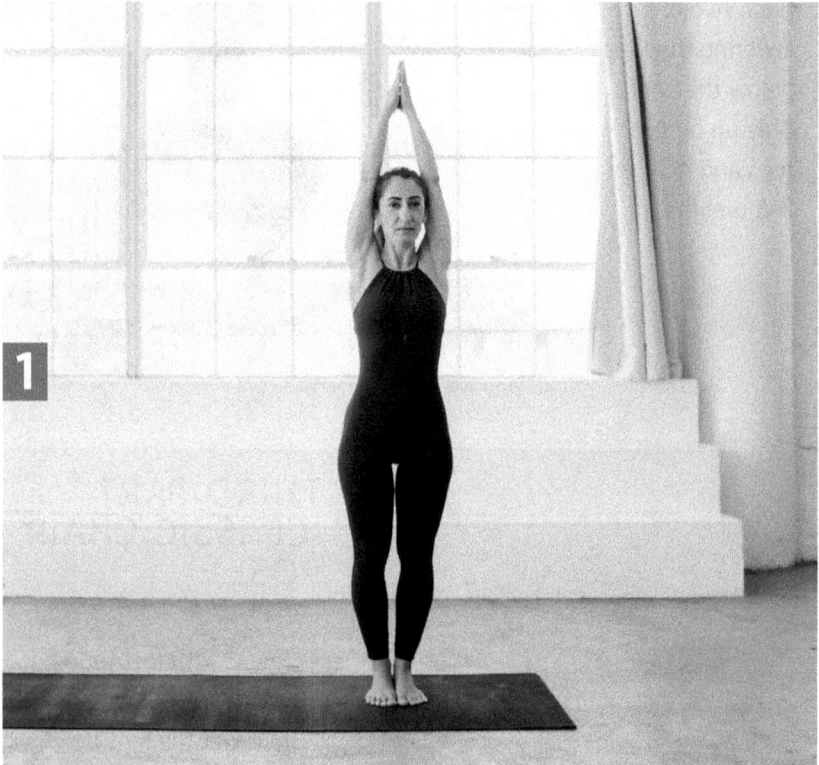

- Start with feet together and arms by your side.

- Inhale and lift the arms up overhead.

- Exhale and simultaneously cross the right arm under the left, wrap the arms once or twice around and bring the palms together.

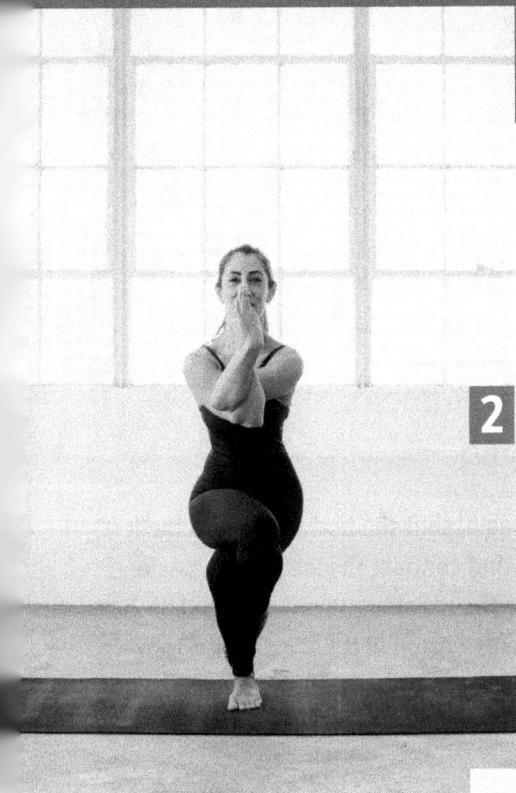

- Inhale and on the exhale, lower the hips and lift the right leg over the left.

- Eliminate any gap between the arms and legs to create compression.

- Bend knees to bring hips as low as possible but avoid bringing the hips below the level of the knees. Actively pull the elbows down to create stretch between shoulder blades and upper back.

2

- Ideally align wrists, elbows, knees and ankles in one vertical line. Hold for 3–5 breaths.

Repeat on other side.

3

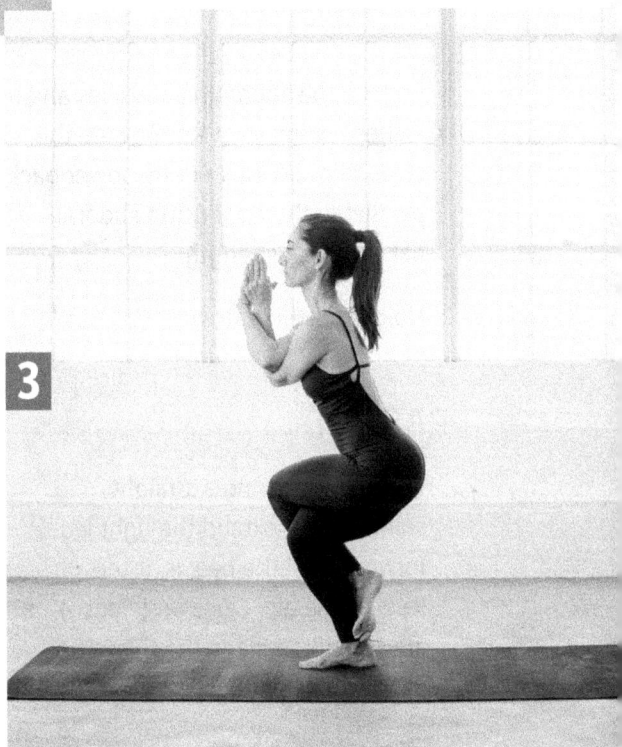

6. Standing Head-to-knee Pose

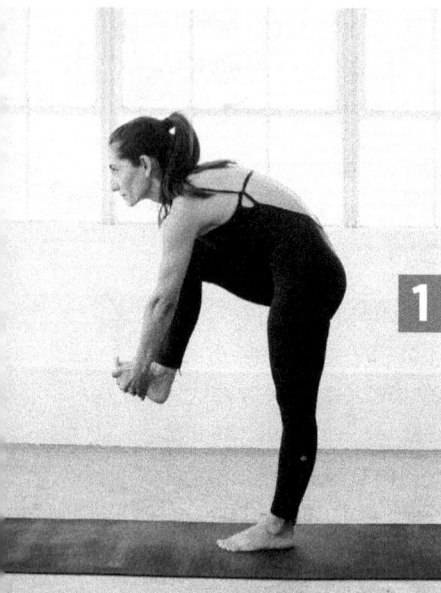

Standing head-to-knee pose helps to build strength, balance and mental focus. This pose strengthens the ankles, legs, hips, abdominal and back muscles.

PART I

- To begin, shift the body weight to the left foot and contract the left thigh muscle. Keep the leg straight with no bend or hyperextension in the knee joint. From the side view, intend to keep the hip, knee and ankle joint in a vertical straight line.

- Engage the abdominal muscles and round over to hold the right foot 2 inches behind the toes. Be sure the foot being held is light in the hands so as to avoid strain in the lower back. Ideally the right thigh is held parallel to the floor using abdominal and back strength.

- Hold for 3–5 breaths.

PART II

- While maintaining a straight standing leg, extend the right leg forward until the heel is at the level of the hip. Once both legs are straight, engage the thigh/quadriceps muscles on both legs.

- Hold for 3–5 breaths.

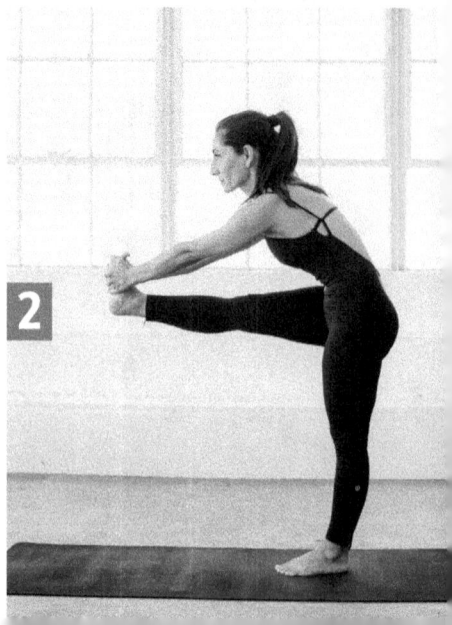

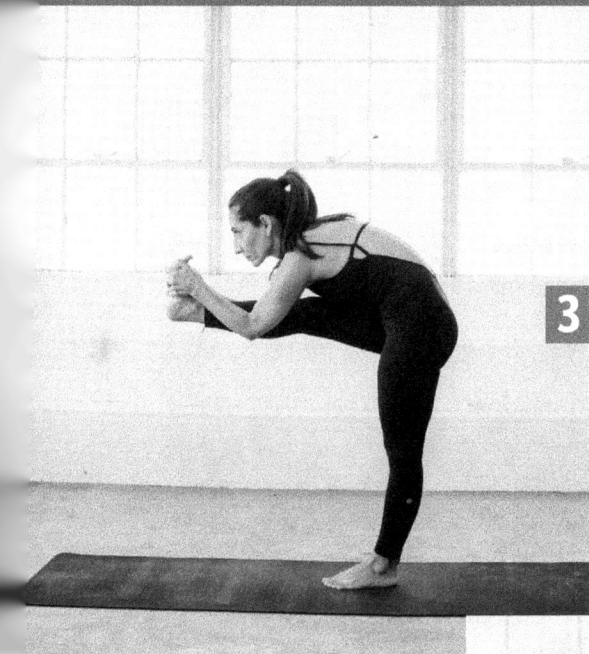

PART III

- Keeping both legs straight and both thighs contracted, bend the elbows toward the floor until elbow points are slightly below the calf muscle.

- Hold for 3–5 breaths.

PART IV

- Maintaining all the above details of the pose, slowly bring the forehead down to touch the knee while continuously rounding the spine.

- Hold for 3–5 breaths.

Repeat on the other side.

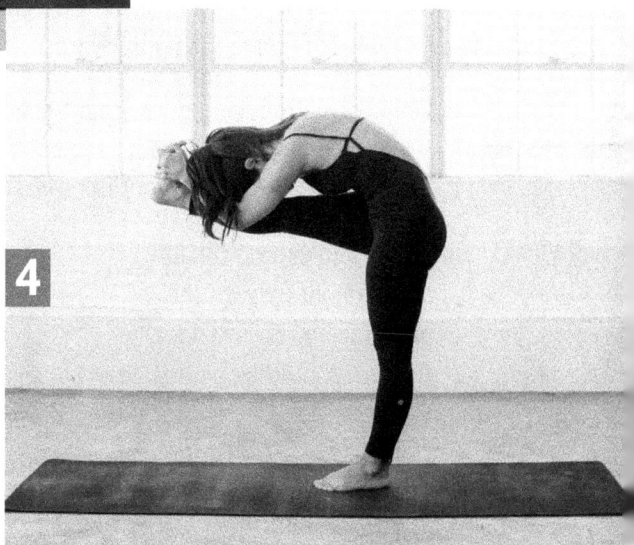

This pose takes tremendous patience. Please master each step before moving on to the next. For example, it is ok to work on Part I of the pose while building strength in the standing leg for months before moving on to Part II. Please do not rush this process. It is one of the most challenging postures.

7. Standing Bow Pose

This pose helps build physical
stamina and mental concentration.
It builds strength in the legs, arms and
back. It also helps improve mobility
in the skeletal structure and joints,
specifically in the areas of the spine,
shoulders, hips and rib cage.

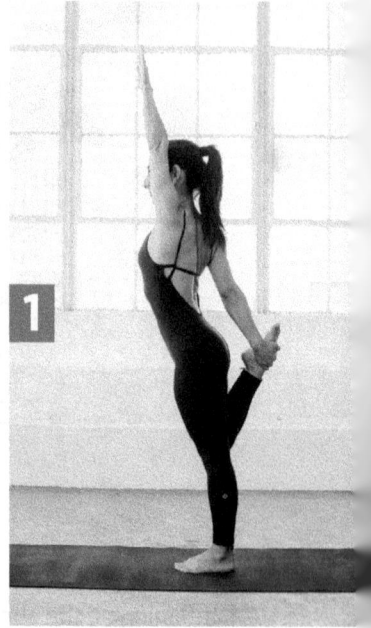

- Begin with feet together and touching.

- Bend the right knee to bring the foot
  back and behind the hip. Grab the right
  foot with the palm facing outward.

- Keep the palm facing out without twist-
  ing the wrist. Grip the foot at the bony
  shelf between the ankle and the toes.

- Inhale and extend the left
  arm straight up with the
  palm facing forward. Ideally
  the arm should be alongside
  the ear.

- Exhale and kick the right foot
  into your hand, away from
  the body and up.

- Bring the torso down until
  the chest and stomach are
  parallel to the floor.

- Hold for 3–5 breaths.

Repeat on the other side.

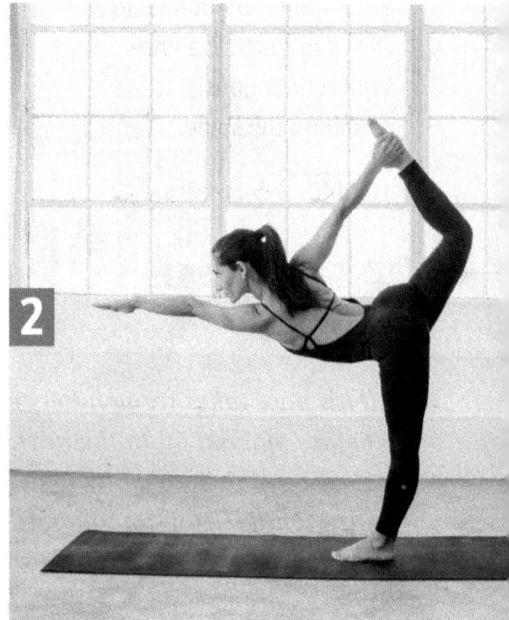

8. Balancing Stick Pose

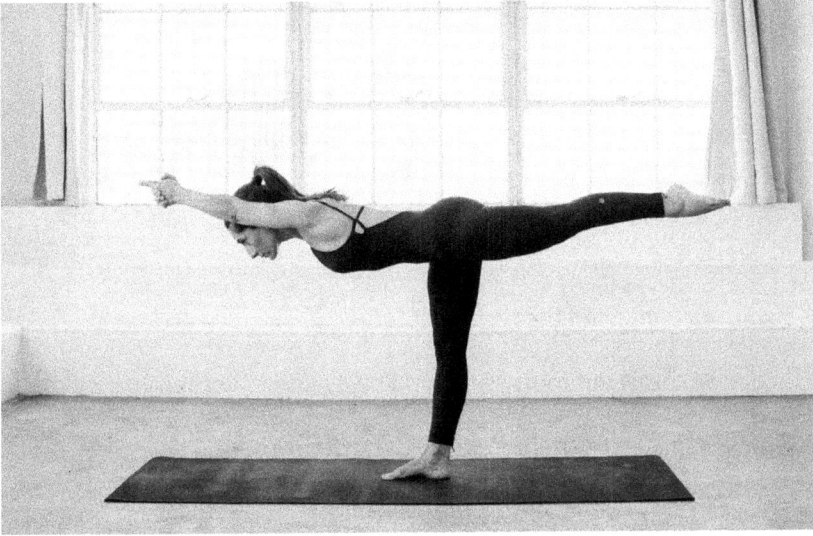

This pose elevates the heart rate and benefits the cardiovascular system. It improves the mobility in the shoulder and hip joints while strengthening arms and shoulders, legs, back and abdominal muscles.

- Begin standing with the feet together.

- Inhale the arms up overhead and step forward onto the right foot.

- Exhale and bring the chest down and the leg up until everything but the standing leg is parallel to the floor. Gaze 4 feet ahead, keeping the arms touching the ears/head.

- Hold for 3–5 breaths.

Repeat on the other side.

The goal in this pose is to keep arms and legs perfectly straight. This is the primary step before working on getting the entire body parallel to the floor.

9. Standing Separate Leg Stretching

This pose helps to stretch the back of the legs and the spine. It is an inversion pose which means the head is below the heart. This pose lowers the heart rate and improves blood flow to the brain and endocrine glands. It also builds strength in the arms and legs.

- Begin standing with the feet together.

- Inhale the arms out to the sides and up overhead to touch the palms.

- Exhale and step the right foot out to the right about 4 feet.

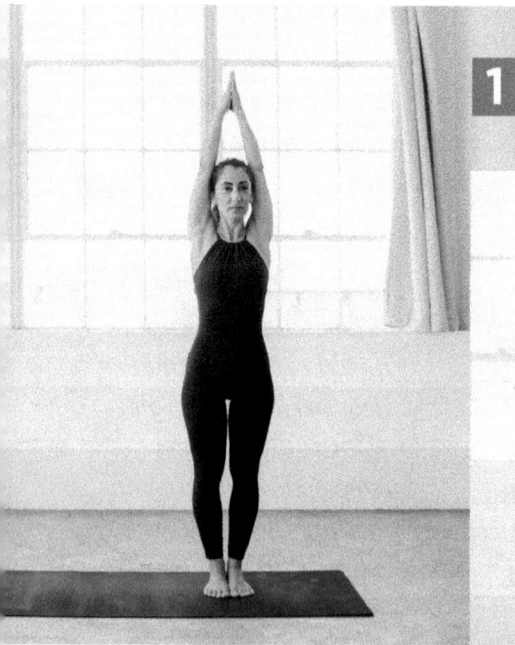

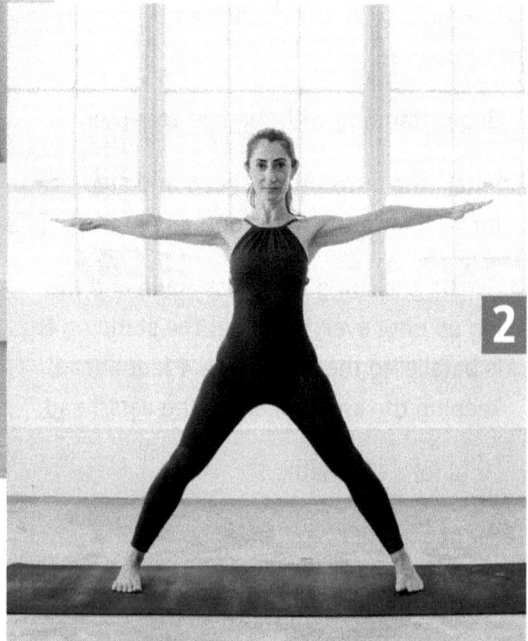

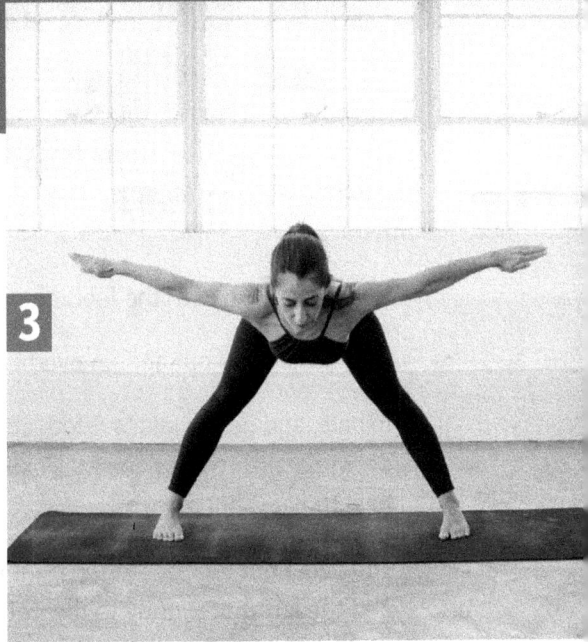

- Inhale and on the exhale, bend forward at the hip joints, keeping arms, legs and spine in straight positions. If there is weakness or discomfort in the back, place the hands on the hips to bend forward.

- Grab the heels. If the heels cannot be reached, place the palms on the floor with fingertips aimed forward.

- Straighten the legs and gently pull with the arms. Aim to touch the forehead to the floor between the feet. Eventually aim to touch the crown of the head. The goal is to keep the legs straight and eventually create a straight spine.

- Hold for 5 breaths.

- Move out slowly while breathing to avoid dizziness.

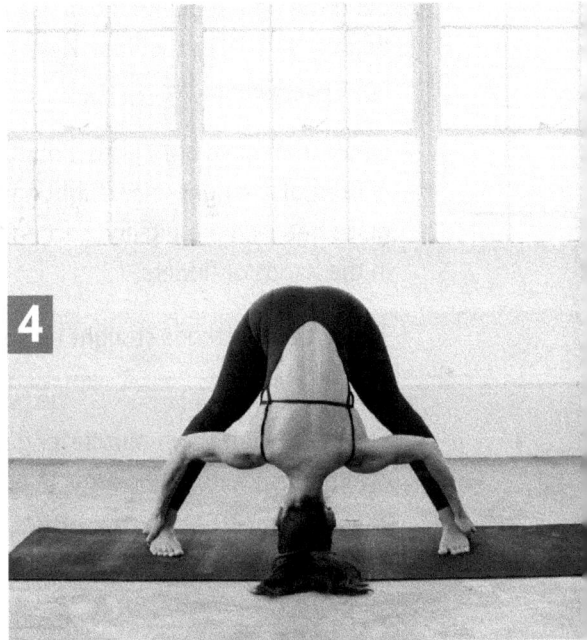

10. Triangle Pose

Triangle pose helps to activate all muscles of the body and improves flexibility in the hips, shoulders and spine. This pose also strengthens the legs, arms, abdominal and back muscles.

- Begin standing with the feet together.

- Inhale the arms out and up overhead, and touch the palms.

- Exhale, and gently take a 5-foot step to the right. Bring the arms down parallel to the floor. Make sure heels are in the same line; heel to heel alignment.

- Turn the right foot out to the right until it's parallel to the mat and the left foot slightly to the right as well, so as to keep the knee safe.

- Bend the right leg until the hips are in line with the knee and the thigh is parallel to the floor. Keep the right knee directly over the right ankle joint.

- Inhale and move both arms simultaneously. Bring the right elbow in front of the right knee. Right hand extends so the fingertips graze between the big and second toe. Avoid placing body weight in the hands or fingers.

- The left arm extends straight up so that both arms form one vertical line.

- Engage the left thigh muscle, engage the abdominal muscles and continuously extend the arms in opposite directions.

- Hold for 3–5 breaths.

Repeat with the other side.

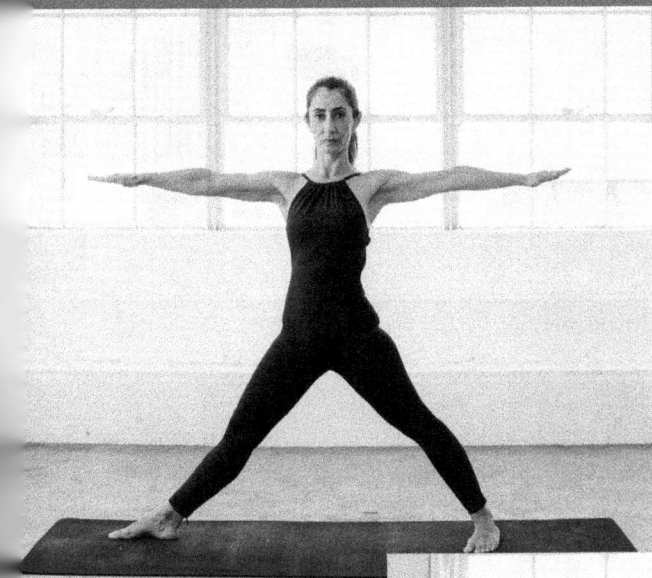

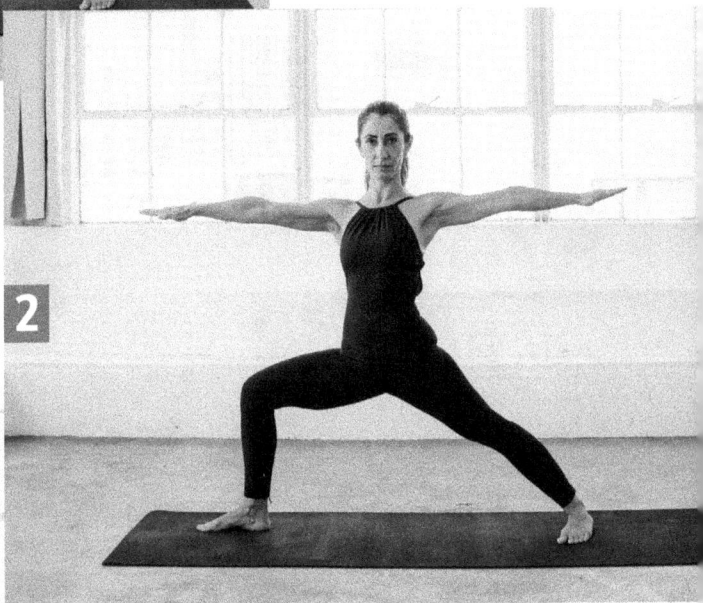

2

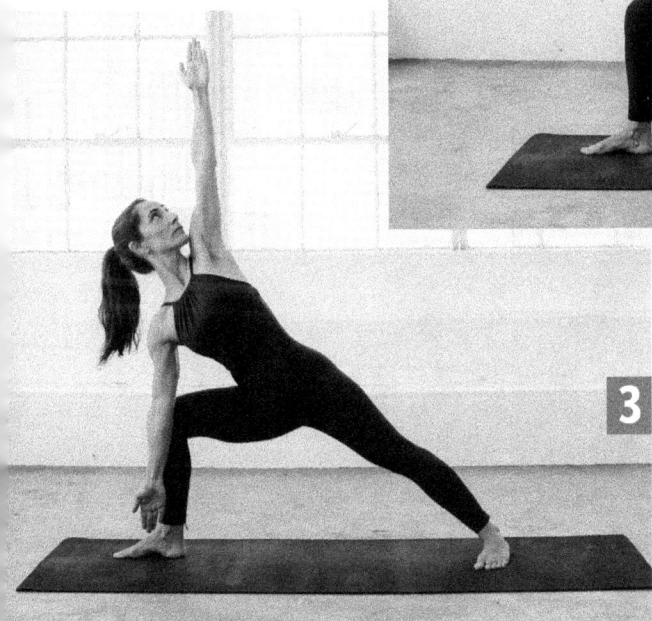

3

11. Separate Leg Forehead-to-knee Pose

This pose stretches the back of the legs, hips and torso including the lower, middle and upper back. It strengthens the abdominal muscles and compresses the thyroid and parathyroid glands, along with stretching the kidneys and adrenals.

- Begin standing with the feet together; toes and heels touching.

- Inhale the arms up overhead to touch the palms.

- Exhale and take a 3-foot step to the right.

- Pick up your toes and rotate on your heels to the right.

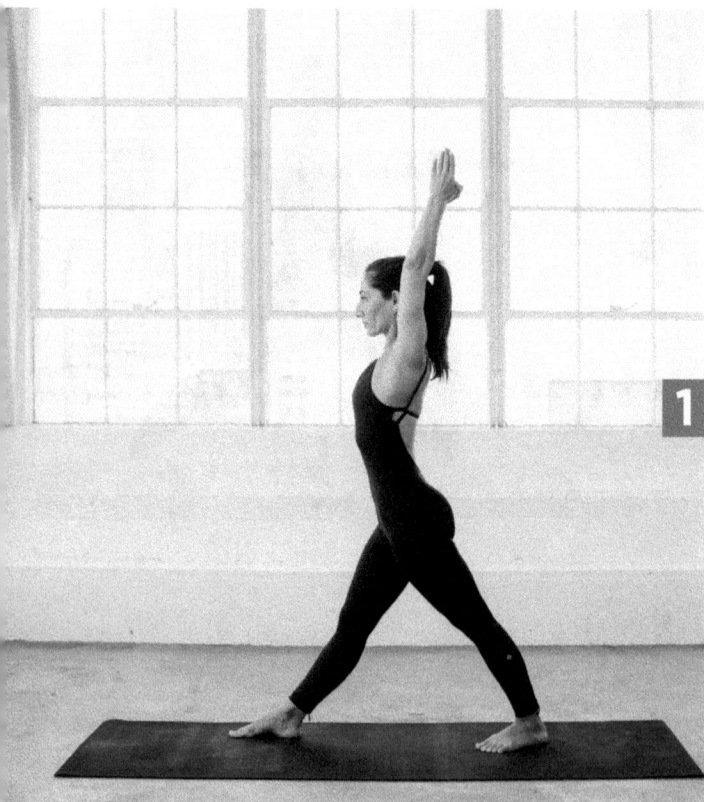

- Make sure the hips are aligned, tighten the abdominal muscles and slowly round down to touch the forehead to the knee. Bend the knee as much as you need to get the connection.

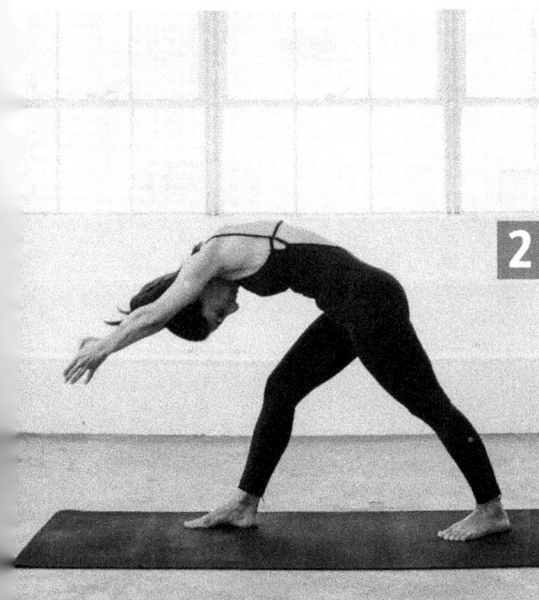

2

- Arms extend forward in straight position and fingertips reach beyond the toes. Keep the palms together unless balance is a challenge. If it is, separate the arms and reach the hands to the floor.

- Gaze at the abdominal area to maintain a rounded spine position.

- Breathing may be challenging due to the compression so focus on small inhalations of breath.

- Hold for 3–5 breaths

Repeat on the other side.

3

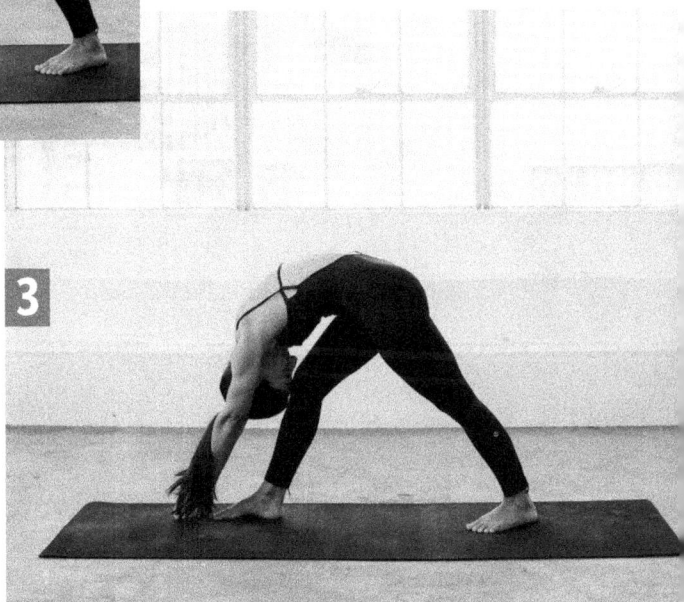

12. Tree Pose

This pose helps to lower the heart rate, maintain hip mobility and reinforce mental focus. Avoid excessive pressure to the knee joints.

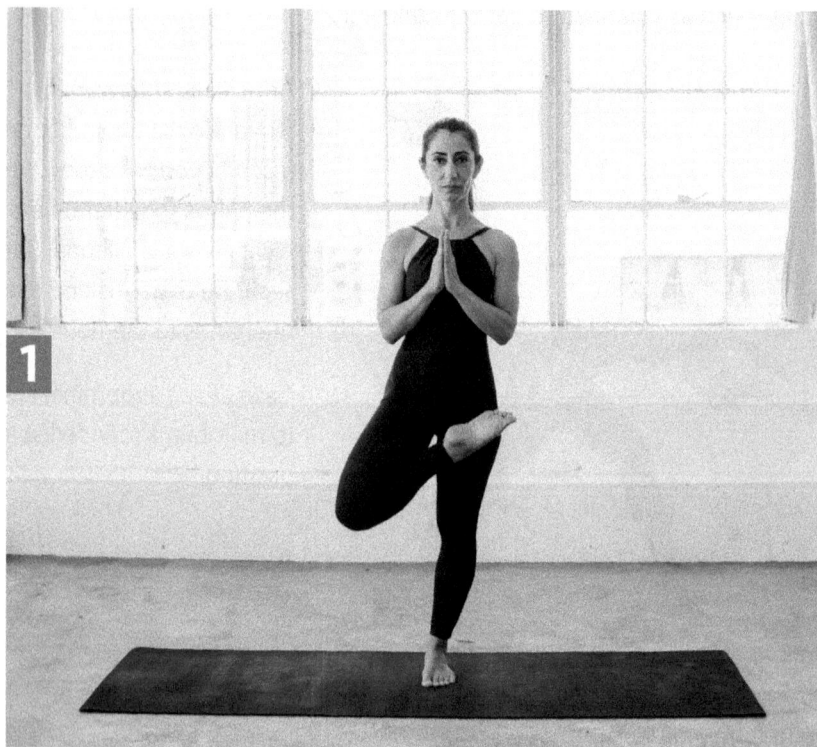

- Begin standing with the feet together.

- Pick up the right foot and bring the knee as high as possible. Bring the foot to the top of the left thigh with the bottom of the foot facing up. Engage the gluteus muscles and gently press the right leg back to externally rotate the hip joint.

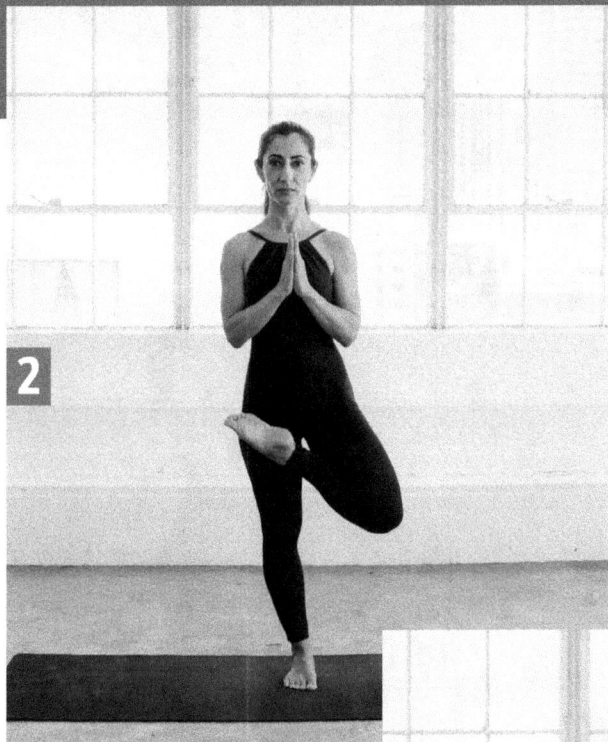

2

- Bring the hands into prayer position with the elbows relaxed alongside the body.

- Hold for 3–5 breaths.

Repeat on other side.

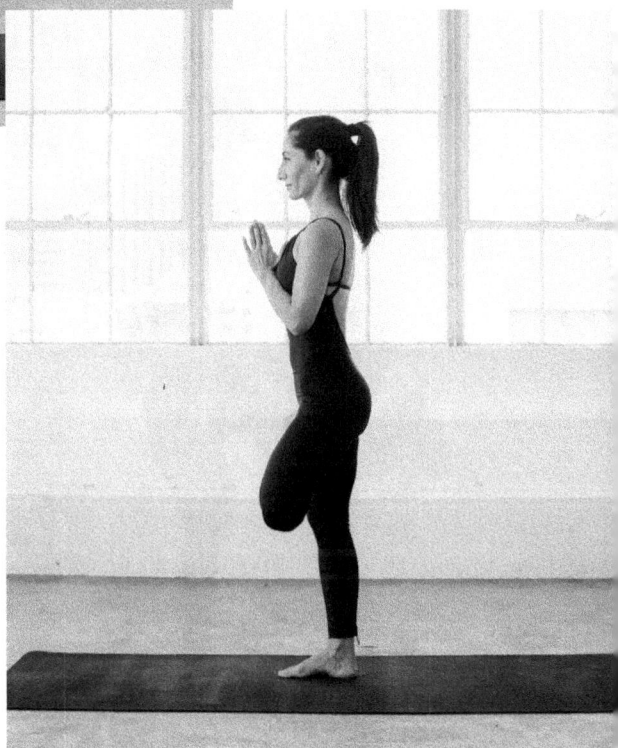

Side view of tree pose

13. Toe Stand

This pose may be a continuation of the preceding pose.

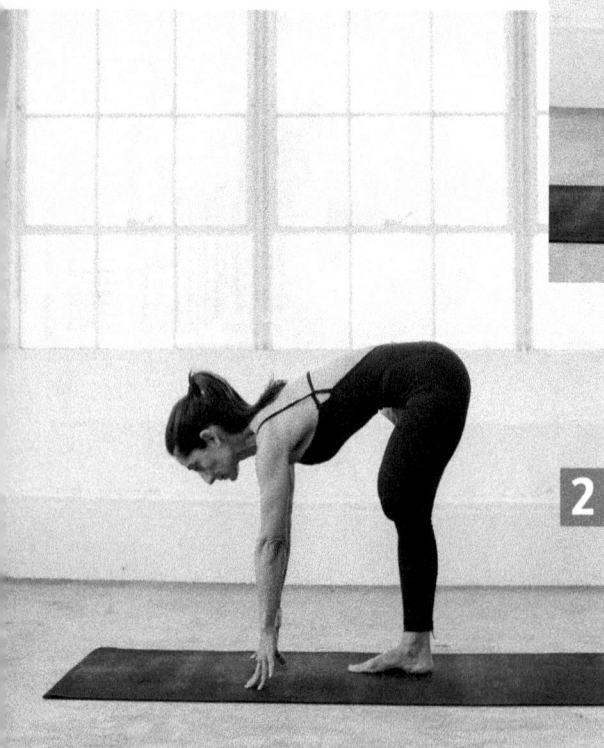

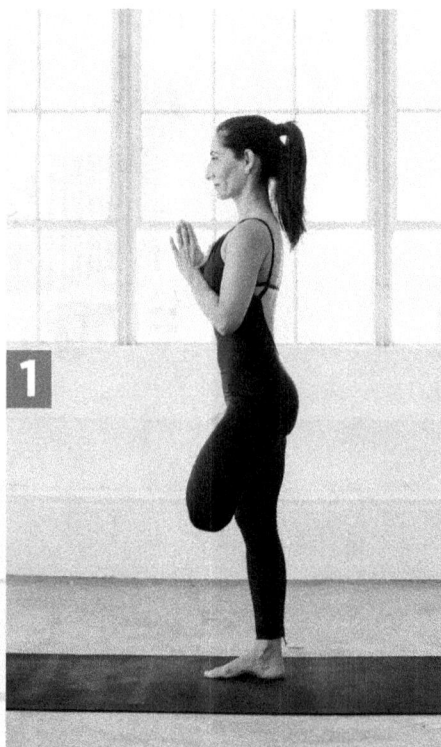

• From the tree pose, shift the gaze to the floor and slowly bend forward at the hips while reaching the hands forward to touch the floor.

Do not do this pose if you are healing from a knee injury.

- Lower the hips down by bending the standing leg. Avoid sitting on the heel; hold hips hovering over the heel. Maintain strength and energy in both legs.

- Slowly bring hands into prayer position.

- Hold for 3–5 breaths.

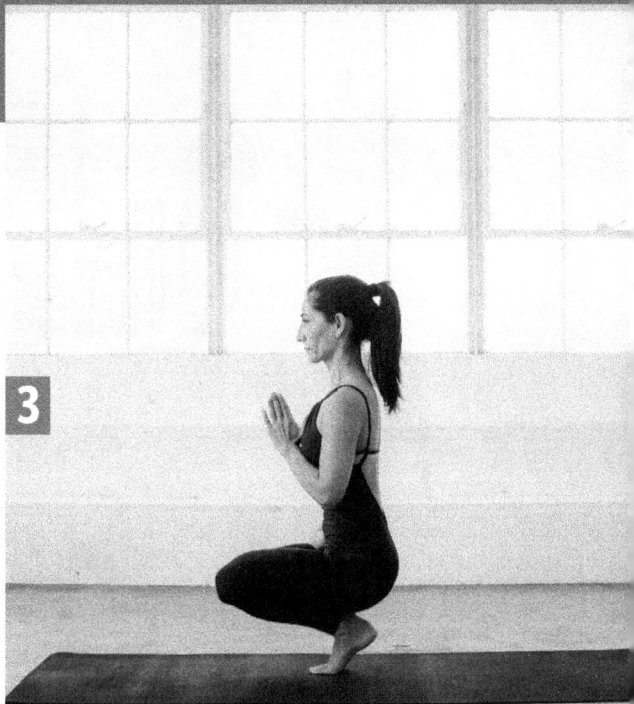

Repeat on other side.

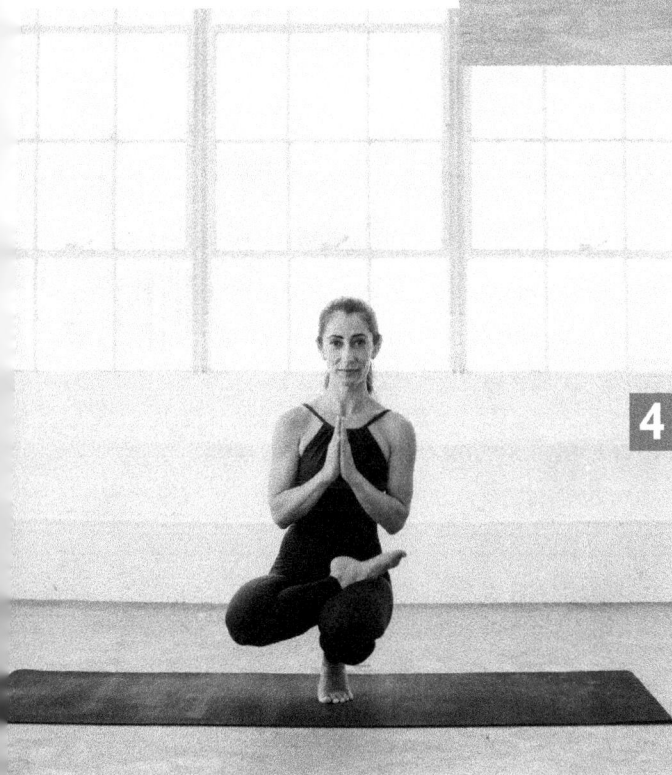

111

14. Savasana or Resting Pose

This pose allows for a rest to lower the heart rate, focus the mind, and practice complete relaxation of all the muscles.

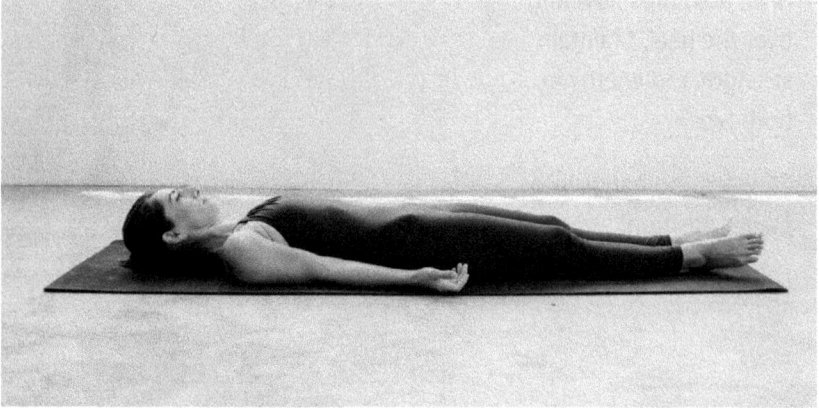

- Lay on your back with the heels touching and the toes outward.

- Arms are alongside the body with the palms facing upward.

- Maintain a soft gaze and observe the movement of the breath.

- This is an ideal pose to practice diaphragmatic breathing. Abdominal breathing allows for the abdomen to move with each inhale and exhale.

Rest for 1–2 minutes and learn to relax and release tension.

15. Wind Removing Pose

This pose helps to mobilize the hip joints and stimulate the digestive system. It also helps to strengthen the arms and the hands along with releasing tension in the neck and back.

- Lying on your back, bend the right leg and grab 2 inches below the right knee with all 10 fingers interlaced.

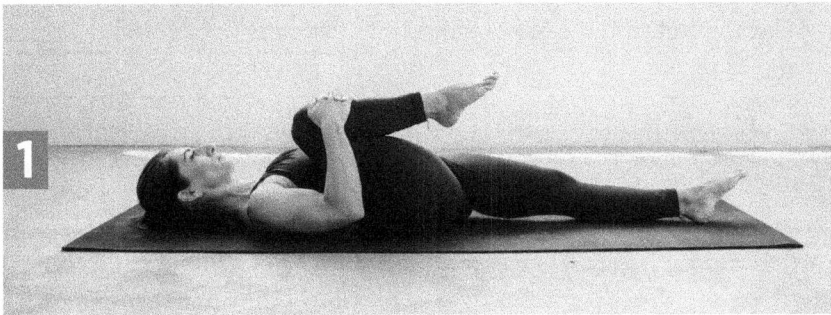

- Be sure to avoid the ribcage as you pull the knee toward the right shoulder and hold for 3–5 breaths.

- Use both arms equally and keep both shoulders on the floor.

- The left leg should remain relaxed with the left calf touching the floor.

Repeat with the left leg, then bend both legs up.

- With both legs up, grab the opposite elbows or high up on the forearms. Keep knees together and pull knees in toward the chest and press the hips down to the floor. Thighs press against the lower abdomen. Avoid pressing thighs against the rib cage.

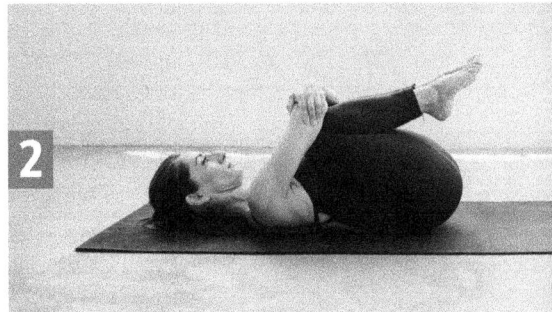

16. Transition Sit-up

This transition pose helps to strengthen the abdominal muscles and stretches the hamstrings.

- Lying on the back, inhale the arms up overhead with the palms facing upward and the thumbs hooked.

- Flex the feet with the toes and heels touching.

- Engage the thighs, gluteus and abdominal muscles.

If you are experiencing back pain, you may bend the legs and grab below the knees and roll forward or simply roll to your side and press up.

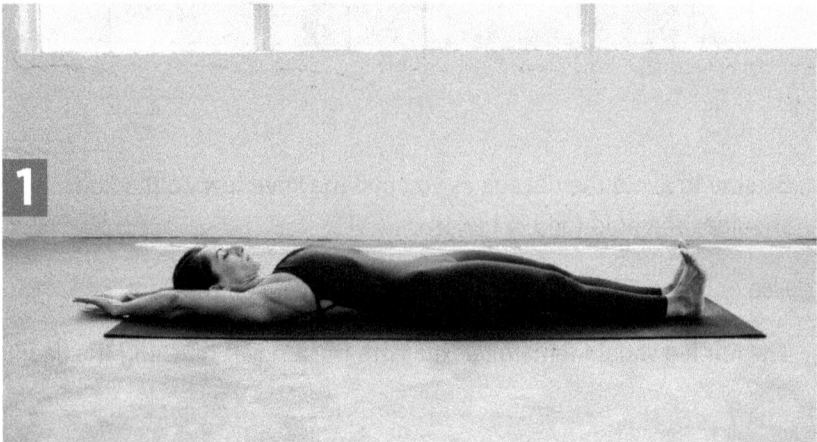

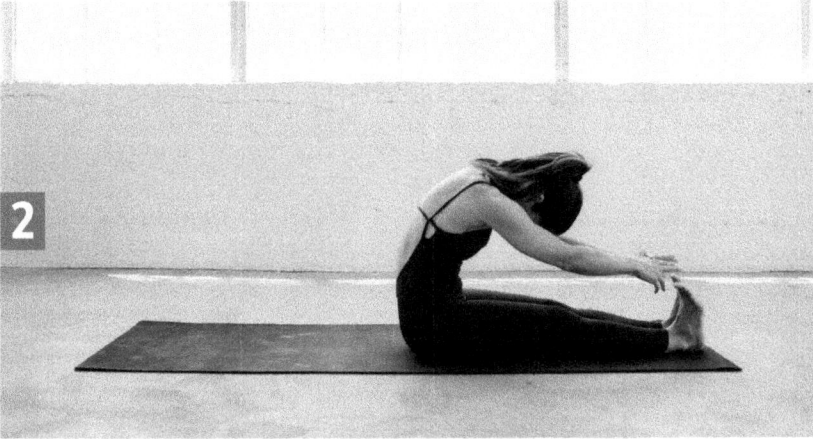

- Sit up with a rounded spine, grab the big toes and exhale 1-2 times.

- If possible, maintain straight leg position with contracted thighs during the term of the sit-up.

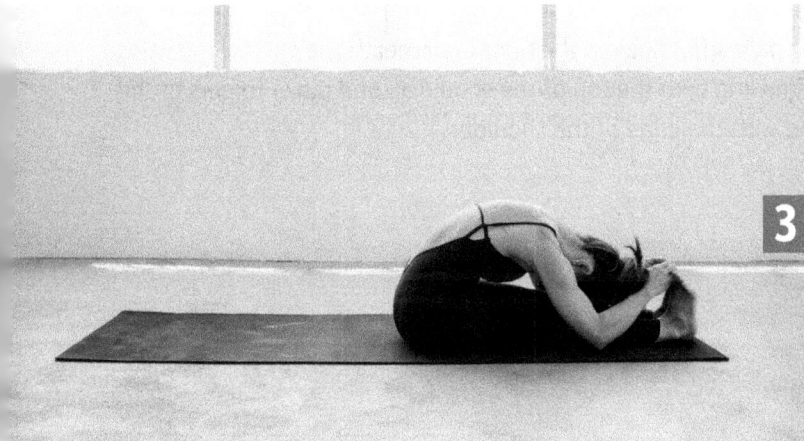

17. Cobra Pose

Cobra pose strengthens the lower back and pelvic floor muscles while creating compression in the kidneys and adrenals. This is a great pose to strengthen and mobilize the entire spine.

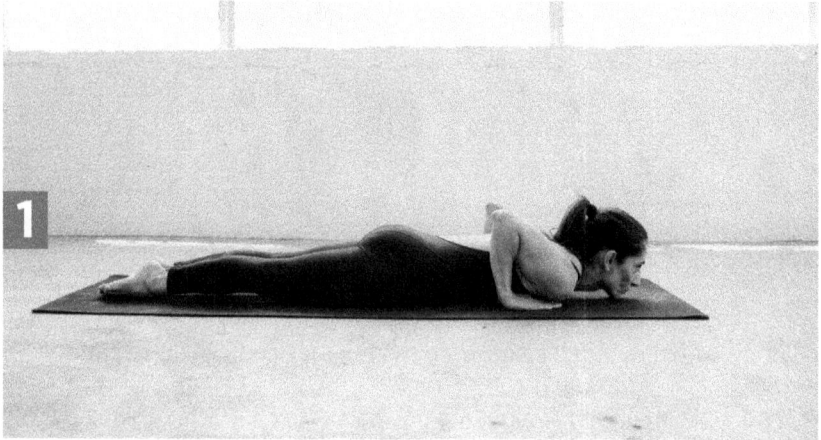

- Start by laying face down.

- Place the palms flat against the floor underneath the chest. Fingertips in the same line with the top of the shoulders and pinky fingers in the same line with the edge of the shoulders.

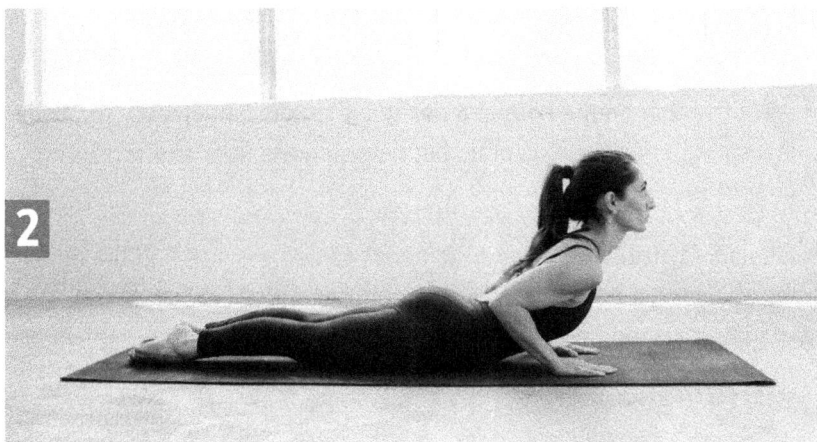

- Engage the leg and gluteus muscles with the feet extended (pointed position).

- Inhale and lift the chest halfway until the arms are in "L" positions. Avoid excessive weight in the hands to use maximum lower back strength. Maintain strong contraction in legs, hips and back. Maintain contact of the feet against the floor.

Between this pose and the next, lying on the stomach, make sure to rest by placing the alternate cheek or ear on the floor, relaxing with arms straight alongside the body and focus on the breath.

18. Locust Pose

Locust pose strengthens the upper back muscles. It also helps to alleviate tension in the neck and upper back and reduce inflammation in the shoulders, elbows, wrists and hand joints.

PART I

- Place the chin on the floor and position the arms underneath the body in a straight position. Maintain flat palms on the floor and spread the fingers out.

- Inhale and lift the right leg up to about 45 degrees, keeping the right hip against the right forearm. Continuously press both hands and shoulders on the floor to shift strength to the upper back.

- Hold for 3–5 breaths.

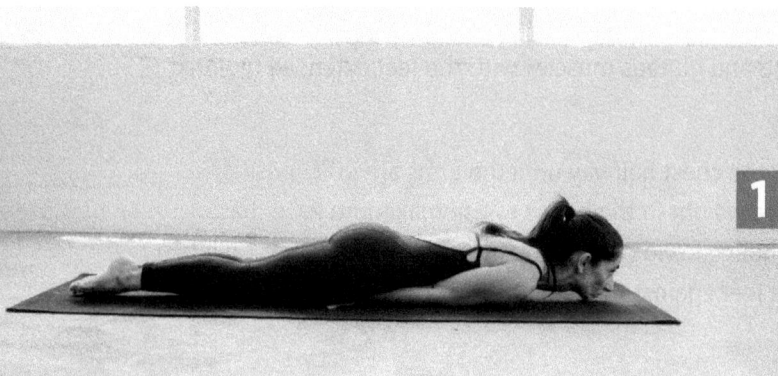

Switch legs and repeat.

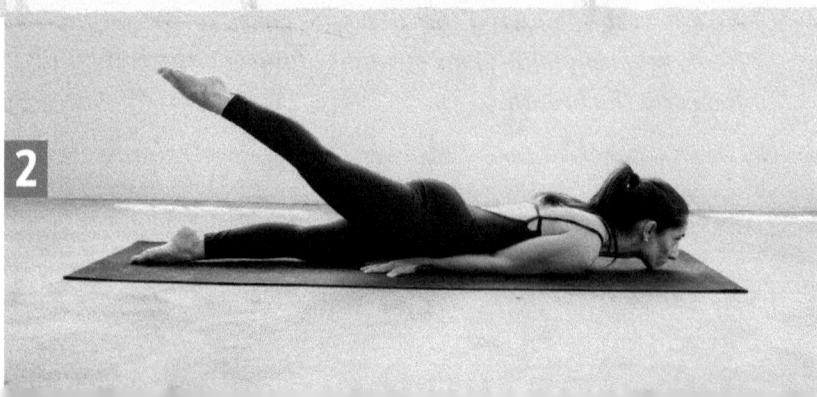

PART II

- Place the mouth against the floor and maintain the position of the head.

- Inhale, engage the gluteus and leg muscles and lift both legs together. Keep the length of the legs together with the knees extended, toes pointed and feet touching.

- Hold for 3–5 breaths.

This pose can be very uncomfortable at first. It is important to have the arms in a straight and full extension (no bend in the elbows) before getting the arms fully underneath the body.

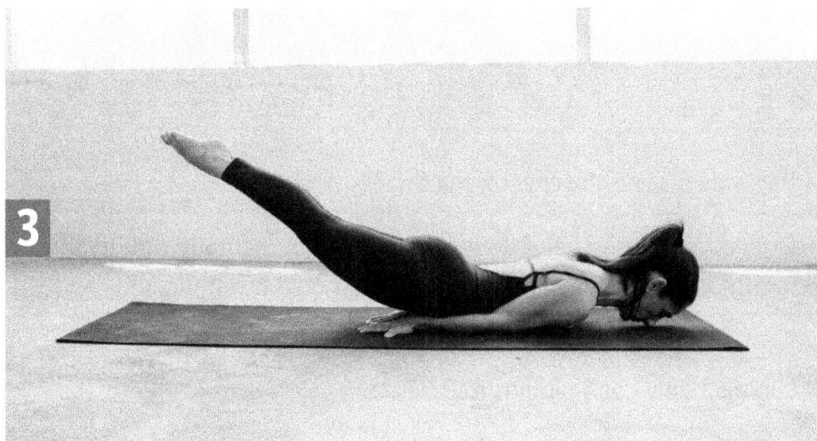

Between this pose and the next, lying on the stomach, make sure to rest by placing the alternate cheek or ear on the floor, relaxing with arms straight alongside the body and focus on the breath.

19. Full Locust Pose

Full Locust pose strengthens the back muscles targeting the middle region along with building strength to the gluteus, arm and leg muscles.

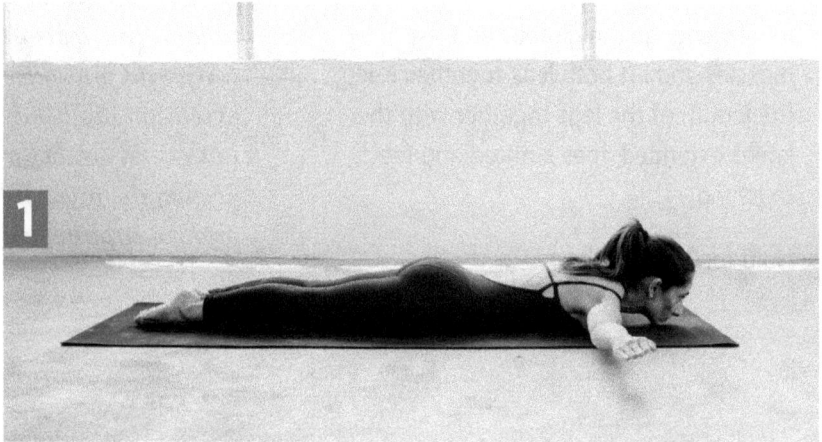

- Begin by placing the chin on the floor.

- Extend both arms straight out to either side of the body with palms facing down and fingers together. Arms should be strong and contracted.

- Engage the leg and gluteus muscles.

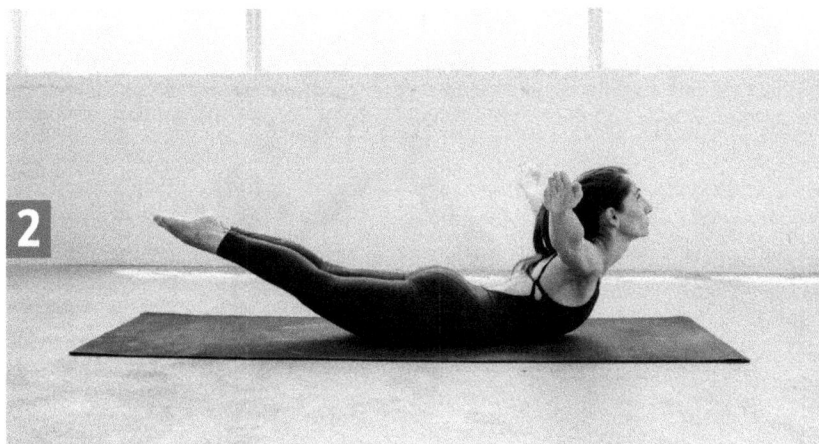

- Inhale and simultaneously lift the arms, legs and chest.

- Keep the length of the legs together with knees extended and hold for 3–5 breaths. Slowly lower down.

Rest.

Between this pose and the next, lying on the stomach, make sure to rest by placing the alternate cheek or ear on the floor, relaxing with arms straight alongside the body and focus on the breath.

20. Floor Bow Pose

Floor Bow helps build and maximize strength in all parts of the back. It creates flexibility and mobility in the spine and opens the rib cage, shoulder joints and hip joints.

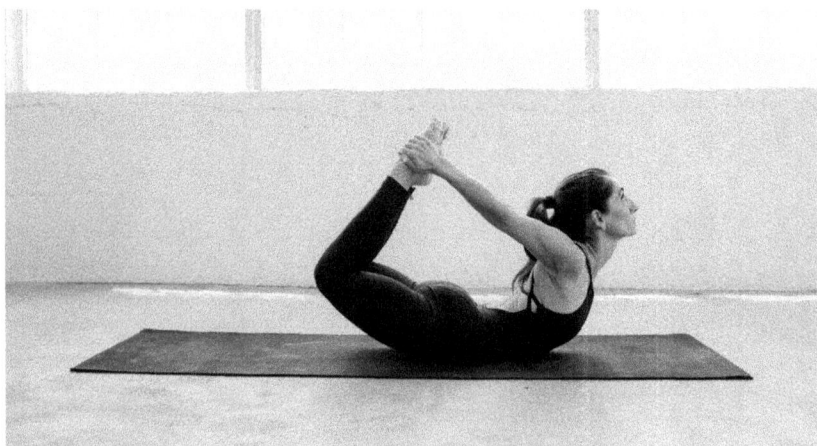

- Place the chin on the floor.

- Bend both legs and grab the feet from the outside, halfway between the toes and heels.

- Begin with knees hip-width distance.

- Engage the gluteus muscles.

- Inhale and actively kick the legs back and up while gazing upward.

- The body weight is on the belly and between the hips and rib cage.

- Avoid body weight pressure on the ribs or hips.

- Hold for 3–5 breaths.

Rest.

21. Child's Pose

Child's pose is a relaxing pose that lowers the heart rate and neutralizes the spine.

- Place the palms underneath the chest.

- Press the body off the floor and into tabletop position.

- Bring the big toes together and open the knees.

- Place hips on the heels and extend the arms forward.

- If the shoulders are tight, rest the arms alongside the lower body with knees and feet together.

- Hold for 3–5 breaths.

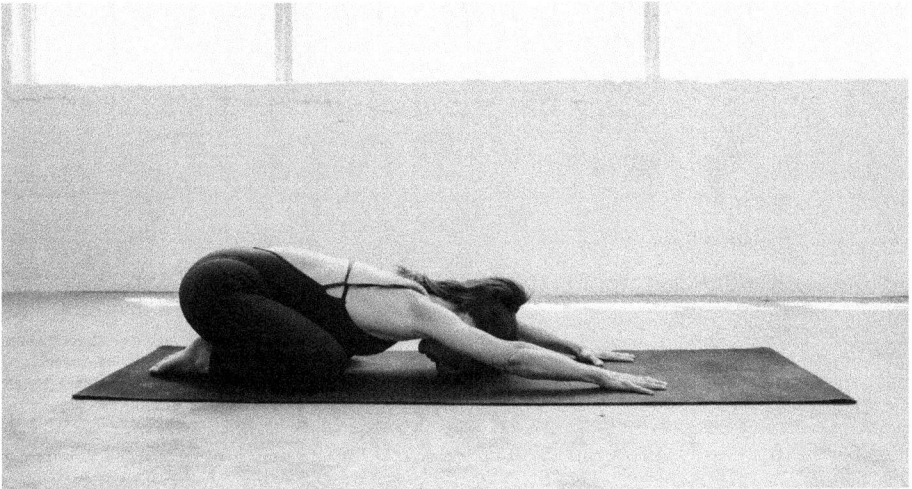

22. Fixed Firm Pose

Fixed firm pose stretches the ankles, knees, thighs and hips. Once the upper body is in contact with the floor, the abdominal and shoulders benefit with a deeper stretch.

- Start with the knees together and stand up on the knees. If you are experiencing knee pain or injury, begin with knees apart.

- Place hands alongside the body for support and slowly lower the hips down between the heels. The feet are outside the hips and straight back. Avoid turning the foot inward or outward to prevent strain to the knees.

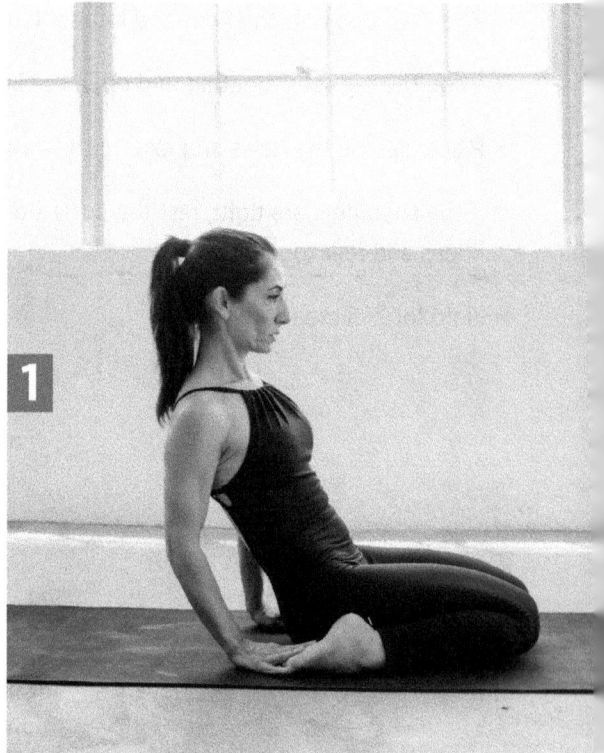

Please work on step 1 before moving onto step 2. The hips must touch the floor before bringing the upper body back. It is imperative that the feet are straight and not turned in or out. Toes and heels must be in the same straight line with the tops of the feet against the floor.

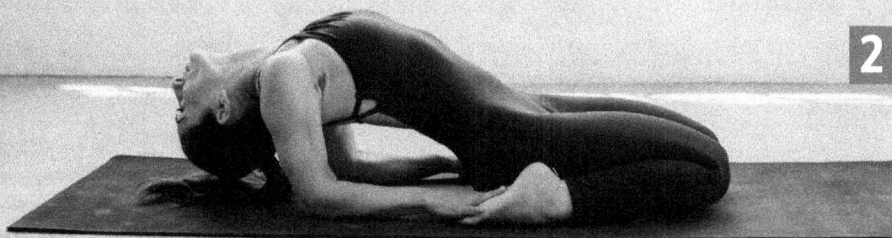

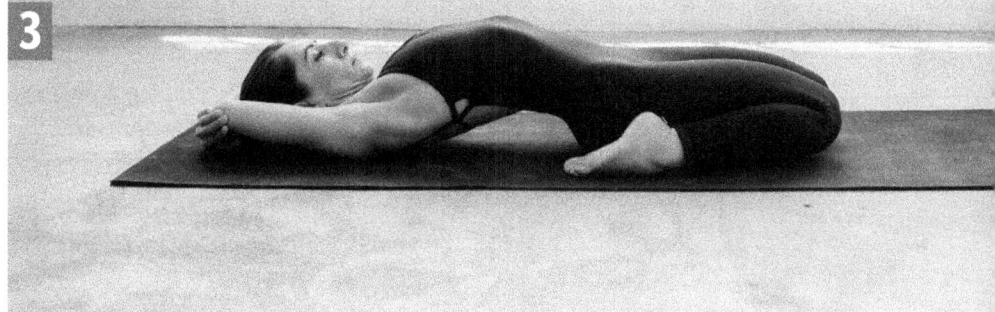

- Once the hips touch the floor, place hands on the feet and slowly lower one elbow at a time. Rest on the elbows and relax the head back.

- Next touch the top of the head to the floor, tuck the chin and place the back of the head on the floor. Once both shoulders reach the floor, extend the arms overhead and grab the opposite elbows.

- Hold for 3–5 breaths.

Rest in Savasana.

23. Half Tortoise Pose

Half Tortoise pose releases tension in the upper back and neck and creates mobility in the shoulders. It stretches the lower, middle and upper back muscles and allows for a slight inversion to move blood flow to the brain. It also stretches the lower regions of the lungs, so make sure to take slow and deep breaths throughout.

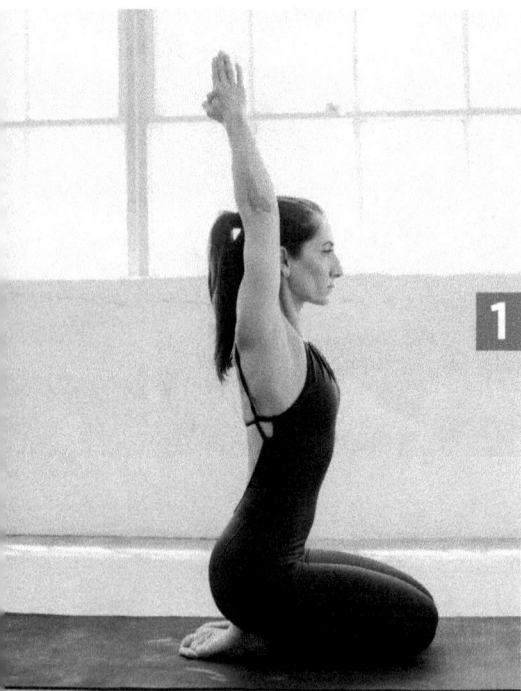

- Start by sitting on your heels with the knees and feet together.

- Inhale the arms up overhead, connect the palms together and cross the thumbs (prayer position).

- Exhale and simultaneously bend forward at the hip joints to lower the forehead gently to the floor and then the hands. If this is not possible, bend the body forward until the hands touch the floor and then the forehead.

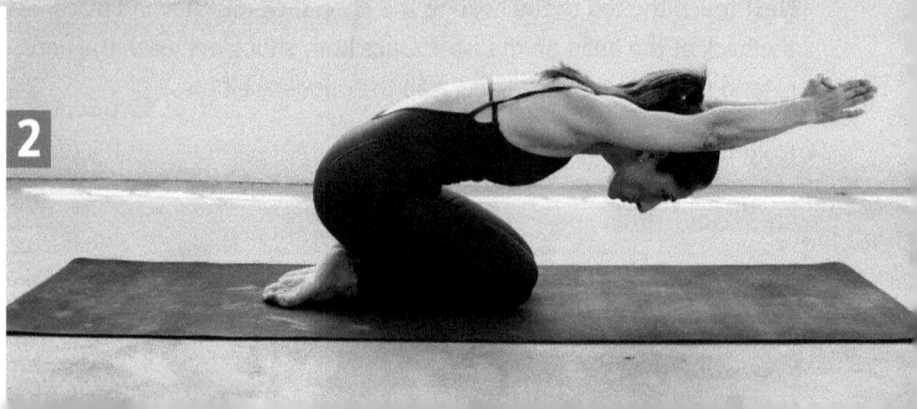

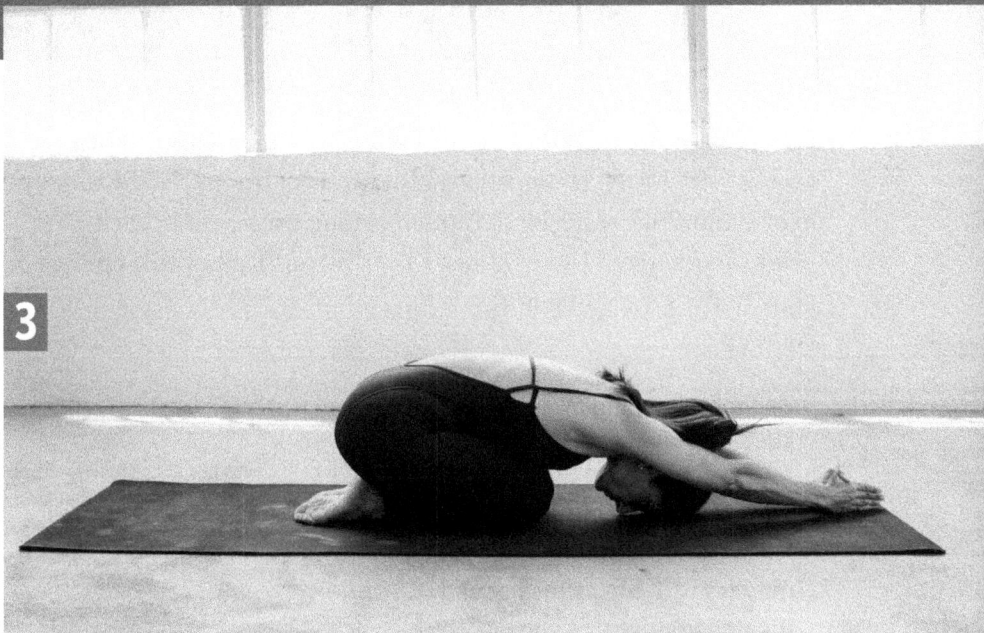

- Try to keep the hips touching the heels, and arms actively stretching forward. The sides of the pinky fingers touch the floor while the wrists, elbows and arms remain off the floor.

- Actively stretch arms forward while simultaneously pressing the hips onto the heels.

- Touch the forehead to the floor and keep the chin away from the chest. This creates a straight line in the spine from upper to lower back.

- Hold for 3–5 breaths.

Slowly come out of the pose and Rest in Savasana.

The goal is to have the hips on the heels and the forehead touching the floor. If neither is possible at first, try to have the forehead touch before working the hips onto the heels.

24. Camel Pose

Camel pose opens the chest and releases tension and tightness around the heart. It helps to maintain mobility in the rib cage, spine, shoulders and hips. Camel pose is the deepest backbend of the sequence. Please do not skip this pose. This will change your body, your spine and your life!

- Begin by standing on your knees. Position knees to hip-width distance.

- Place hands on your gluteus muscles with the palms flat and the fingertips pointed downward. This will help reinforce support and stability.

- Inhale and lift the chest.

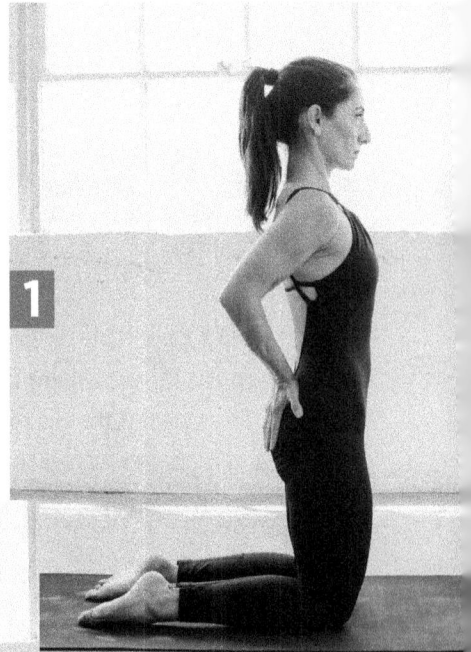

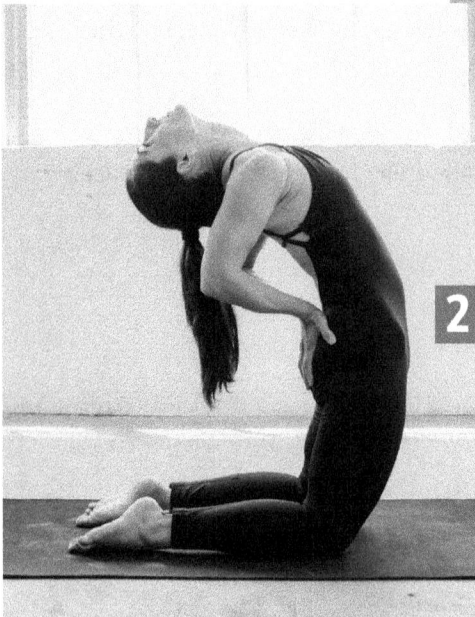

- Exhale and slowly relax the head back while moving into a backbend.

- Hold here for 3 breaths.

- Once the spine has gained flexibility, maintain hip position and slowly reach for one heel and then the other. Once you can hold the heels in the hands, keep the fingertips on the inside of the feet and thumbs on the outside of the feet.

- Be sure to lift up through the chest and avoid collapsing into the lower back. Create an even backbend through the lower, middle and upper back. Keep your eyes open and breathe.

- Hold for 3–5 breaths.

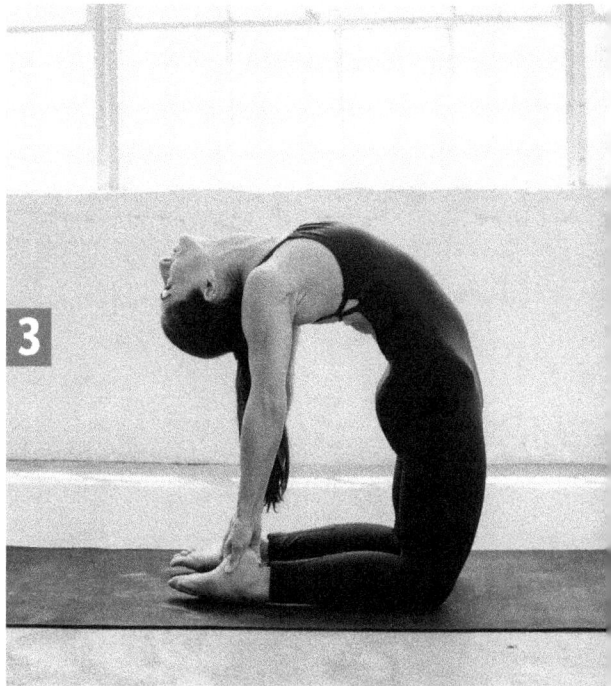

This being the deepest backbend in the sequence, emotions and feelings of dizziness may come up. Don't give up. Keep practicing and your body will soon love the pose.

25. Rabbit Pose

Rabbit pose stretches the back muscles and strengthens the abdominal muscles. It creates compression in the throat to help the thyroid and parathyroid glands along with stretching the kidneys and adrenals. This pose increases blood flow to the brain and helps reduce inflammation of sinuses and congestion.

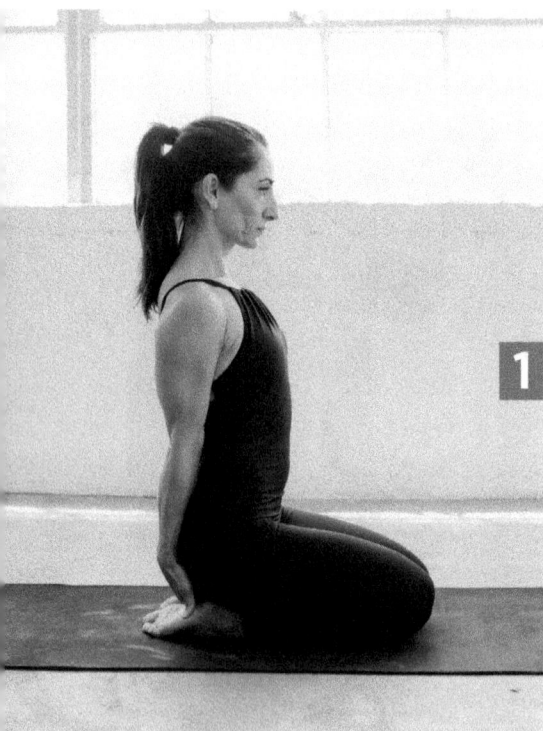

- Begin sitting on your heels with the feet together.

- Grab your heels with the thumbs on the outside and the fingertips on the inside of the feet. **Make sure** you have a secure and tight grip.

Avoid this pose if you suffer from neck pain or herniations in the cervical spine.

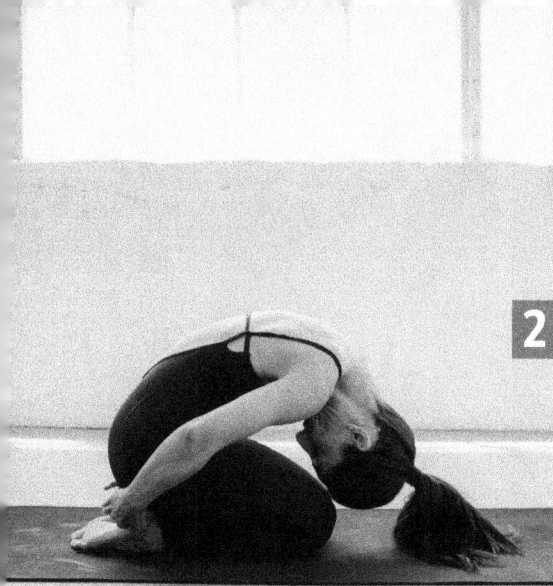

- Contract the abdominal muscles, tuck the chin down to the chest and slowly round your spine and bring the forehead to touch the knees.

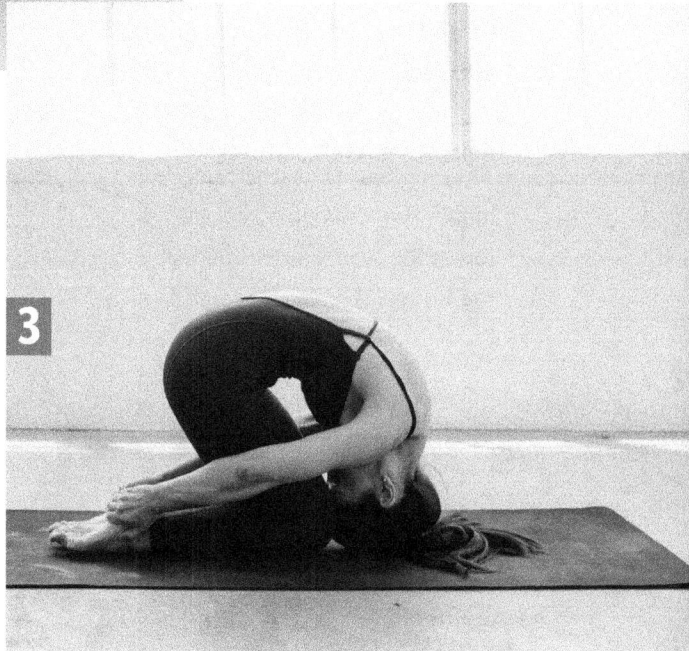

- Slowly lift the hips while simultaneously pulling on the heels. Keep the abdominal muscles engaged and do not place your body weight on the top of the head. Only a slight amount is safe.

- Keep the feet touching while pressing the feet, shins and knees downward against the floor.

- Hold for 3-5 breaths.

- **Important:** Do not turn your head while you are in the pose.

26. Stretching Pose

This pose helps to stretch the back of the legs, align the hips and stretch the spine.

PART I

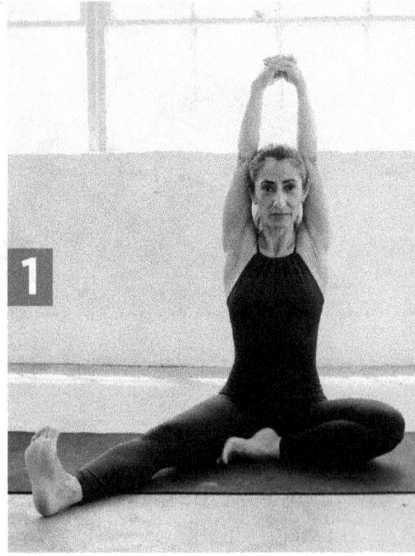

- Begin by sitting down with the legs extended ahead.

- Extend the right leg out at an angle and bend the left leg in, try to touch the sole of the left foot against the right inner thigh.

- Inhale the arms up overhead, touch the palms, and interlace the fingers.

- Turn the upper body towards the extended leg and round the spine.

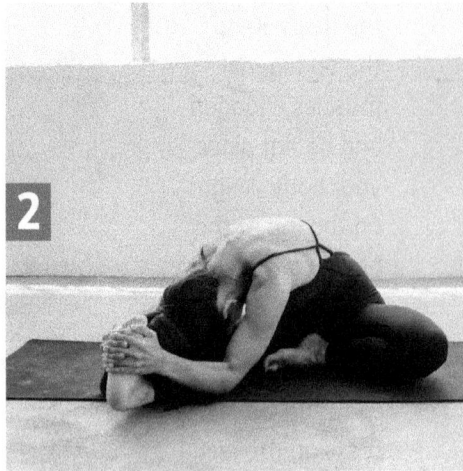

- Grab the foot with fingers interlaced, 2 inches below the toes.

- Bend the right leg as much as needed to create contact with the forehead and knee.

- Eventually straighten the right leg and contract the thigh muscle with the spine rounded. Bend the elbows down to touch the floor.

- Hold for 3–5 breaths.

Slowly round up and repeat with other leg.

PART II

- Extend both legs forward.

- Grab the big toe with each hand using the index and middle finger.

- Inhale and straighten the legs.

- Exhale and stretch the upper body over the legs.

- Create contact with the stomach against the thighs and eventually the chest to the knees.

- Keep the chin up to maintain a straight spine and try to touch the forehead to the toes.

- The goal is to create full hip mobility with straight legs and a straight spine.

- Hold for 3–5 breaths.

Rest in Savasana.

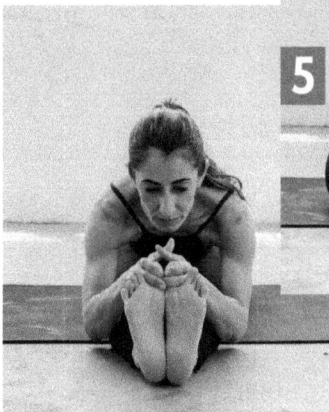

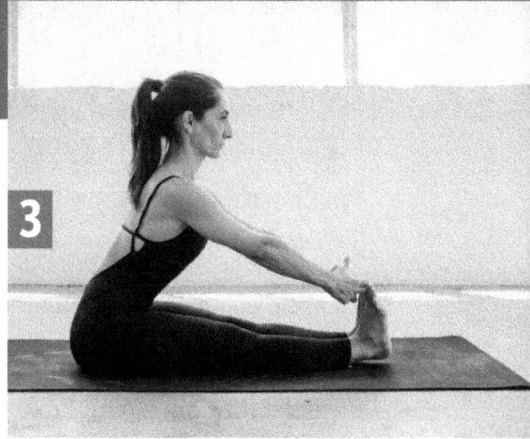

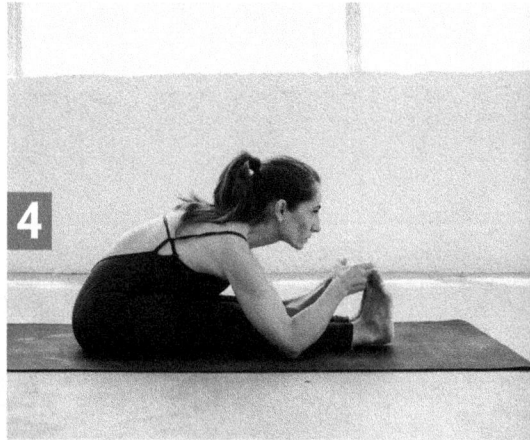

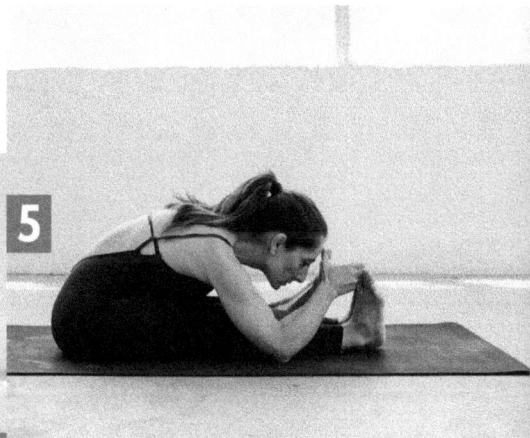

27. Reclined Spine Twist

Reclined Twist helps stretch the lower back and side body. Twists rejuvenate the spine and create mobility.

- Lay on your back and bend the right leg, gently placing the right foot on the left knee.

- Extend the right arm out to the side with the palm at the level of the shoulder.

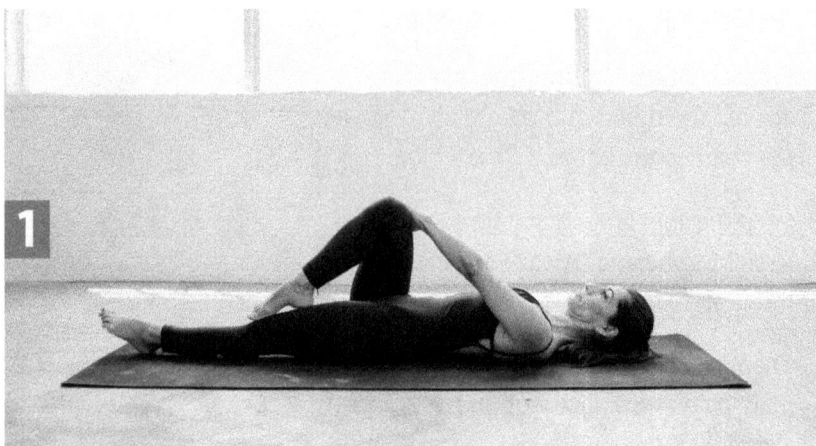

- Place the left hand on the outside of the right knee and gently guide the knee towards the left. For a deeper twist, turn the head to the right.

- Hold for 3–5 breaths.

Repeat on the other side

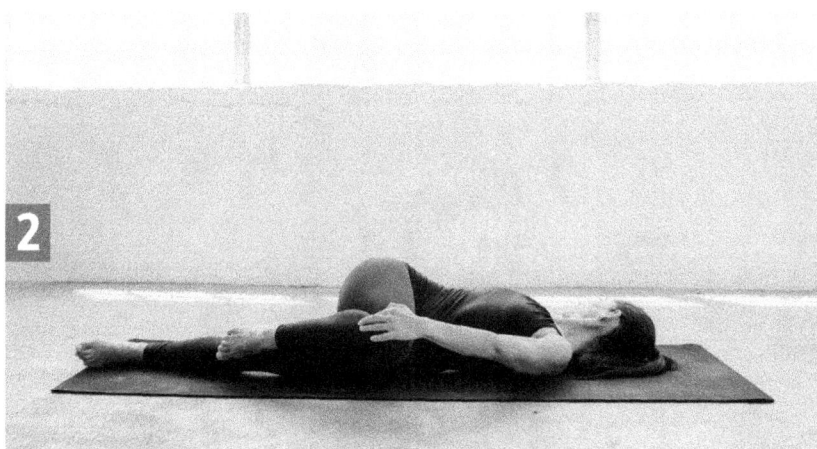

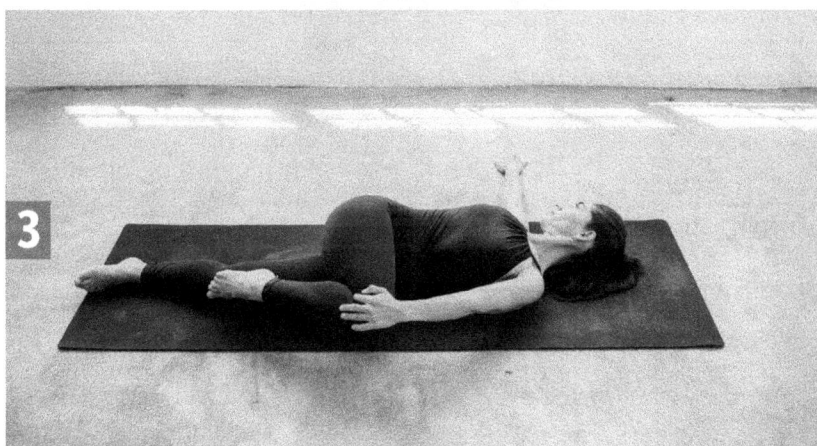

28. Seated Extended Leg Spine Twist

Seated Spine Twist has similar benefits to the reclined twist, yet it reinforces proper hip alignment and creates more stretch to the middle and upper back.

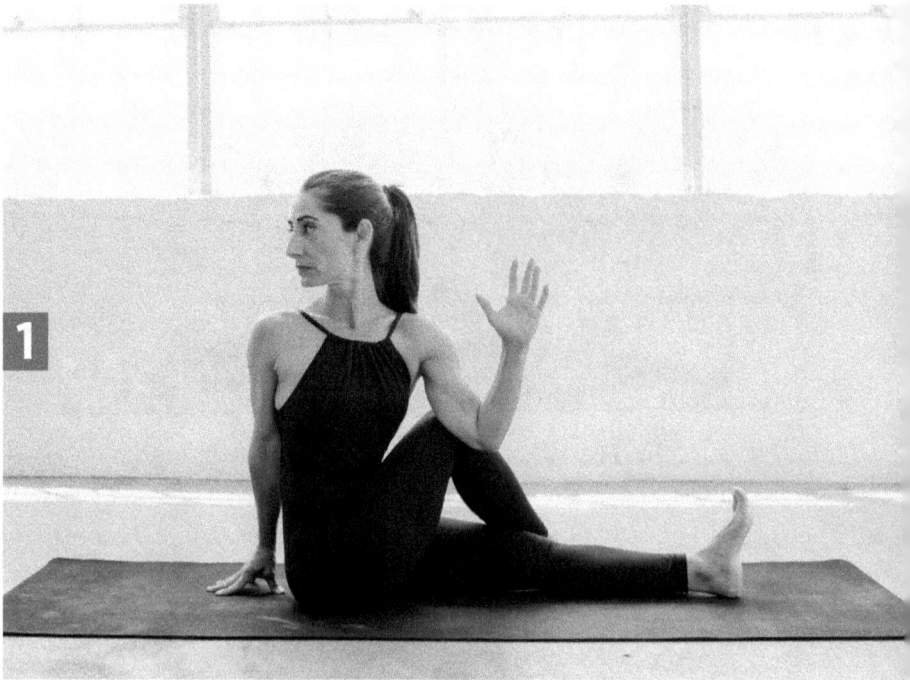

- Begin with both legs extended forward.

- Bend the right leg and place the right foot outside the left knee.

- Place the right arm behind you at the base of the spine. Fingertips are pointed back.

- Extend the left arm up and place the left elbow outside the right knee.

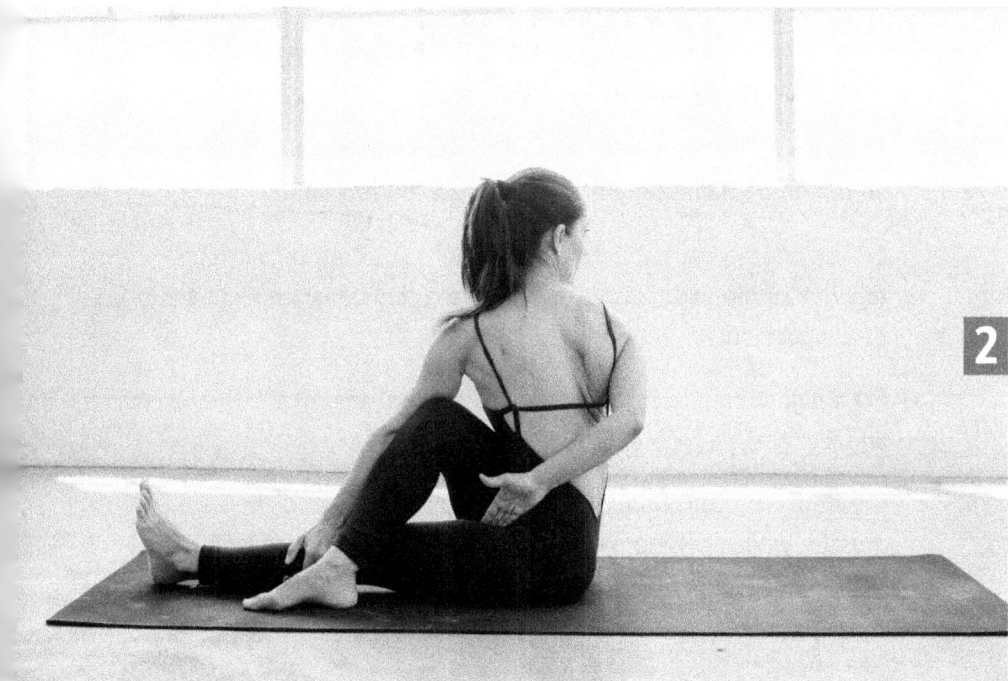

2

- Inhale to lengthen the spine.

- Exhale to twist the spine.

- Hold for 3–5 breaths.

Repeat with other side and rest in Savasana.

For a deeper twist, the arm position can be as shown in photo above.

29. Forearm Plank

Forearm Plank builds strong core muscles: abdominal, back, glutes and pelvic floor. It helps strengthen arms and shoulders and boosts stamina and strength for the entire body.

- Lay on your stomach facing down, and place forearms against the floor, shoulder-width distance apart.

- The safest position for the wrists is to keep hands in fists with thumbs on top or to interlace the fingers with the thumbs on top.

- Extend one leg back at a time in a straight position. Legs can be together or hip-width distance. Toes are curled under and feet are in a flexed position.

- For a higher impact. Place the tops of the feet against the floor so toes and feet are in a "pointed toe" position.

- It is important to continuously engage the gluteus and abdominal muscles while pressing the forearms and fists downward against the floor.

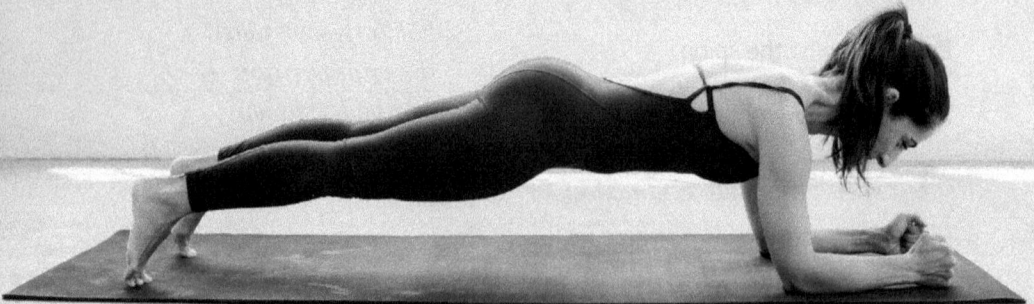

30. Child's Pose

- Place the palms underneath the chest.

- Press the body off the floor and into tabletop position.

- Bring the big toes together and open the knees.

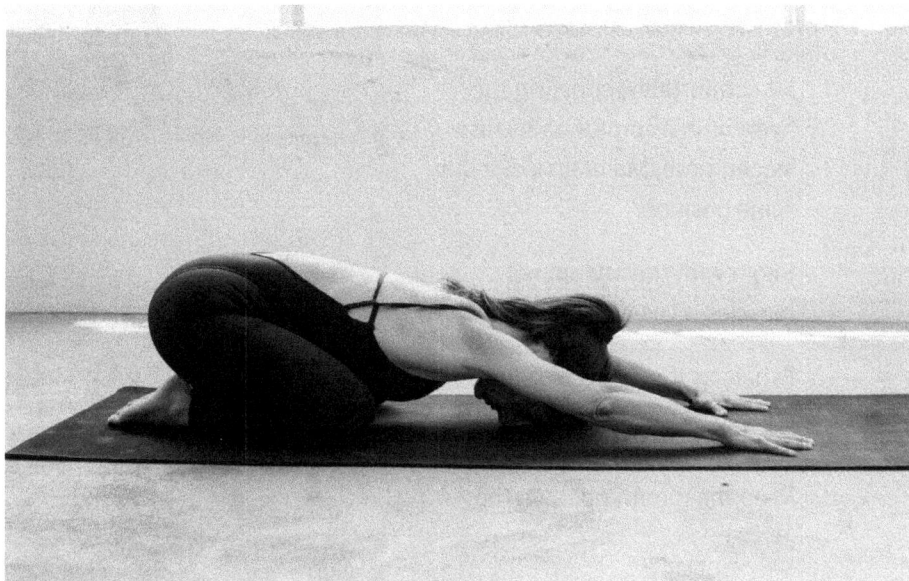

- Place hips on the heels and extend arms forward. If shoulders are tight, bring knees and feet together, relax the head and lay arms alongside the body .

- Breathe deep for 3–5 breaths.

30. Final Breathing: Kapalabhati

Kapalabhati breathing is the "cleansing" breath. Benefits include expelling toxins and free radicals that may form in the lower regions of the lungs. It also strengthens the abdominals and the diaphragm muscle.

- Sit comfortably, either on the heels or in a comfortable cross-legged pose. Maintain a straight spine position.

- Begin with the abdominal muscles relaxed.

- Exhale as if you are blowing out candles and simultaneously contract the abdominal muscles. Keep the mouth open on the exhale.

- Focus on the exhale; the inhale will come naturally.

- Repeat for 60 counts.

- As more experience is gained, learn to do this faster with an even and rhythmic breath pattern known as Bastrika breathing.

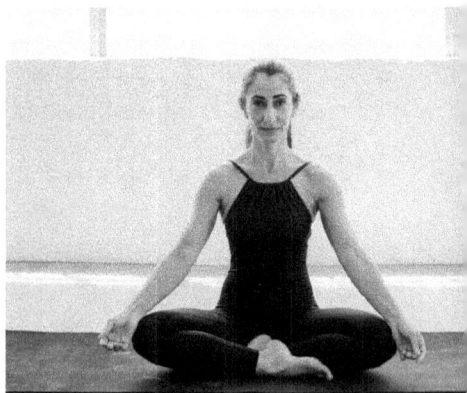

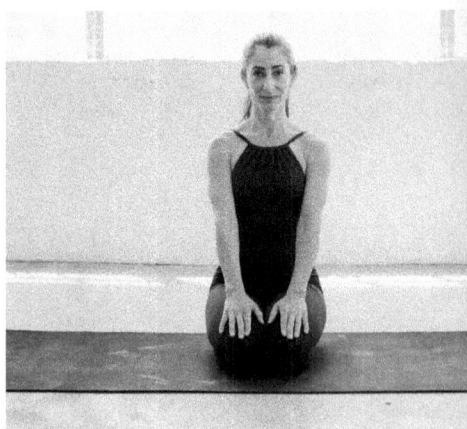

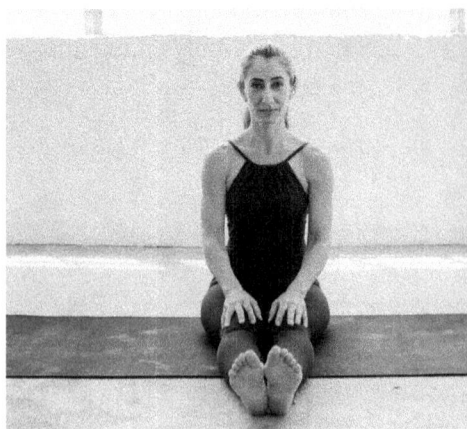

Final Savasana

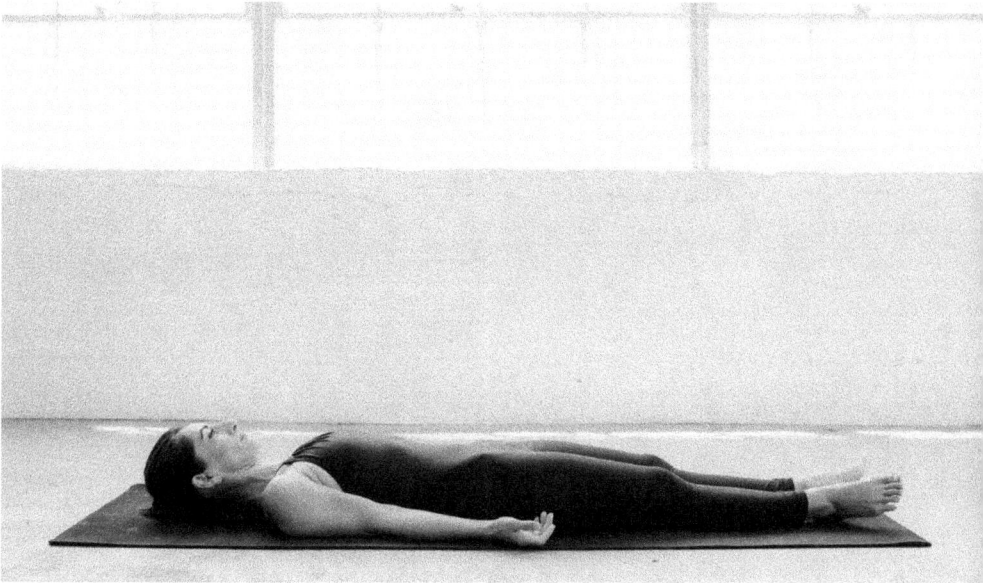

A savasana, as described in pose 14, is strongly encouraged after a practice session. Allow the heart rate to come down, and enjoy the sensations of calm, balance and energy return to the body. Rest for 1-5 minutes to allow all the benefits of your practice to permeate.

Rest into the space and the silence. Feel the deeper self, the wise self, the witnessing presence. At the end of your Savasana, reinforce positive thoughts, prayers, wishes and let them sink in. Love yourself, love the people around you, every living being, and move forward with awareness, a clear mind and an open heart.

A common Sanskrit term to end a practice with is *Namaste* which translates to "I bow to you and recognize the divinity, the Self in me, is the same in All."

This is the way to lasting peace . . . This is *HOME*.

Acknowledgments

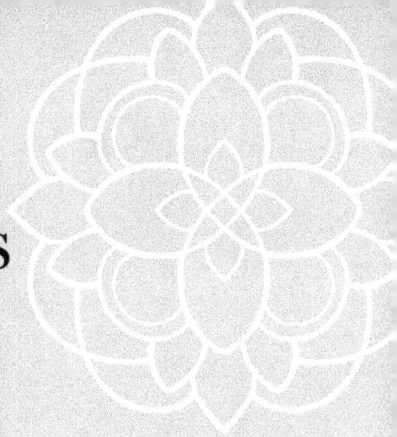

I would like to thank my Mom, who has been my unwavering support throughout my life. She has been my rock and has shown me unconditional love. I would like to thank my Dad for being such a great example of courage, grit and moving forward in the face of fear.

I would also like to thank my niece Sofia Ruhr for contributing her talents with the designs of the mandalas used throughout the book and journal, and a special thanks to Linda Morris for helping me fine tune the additional chapters. I would also like to thank and acknowledge my editor and book designer Michelle M. White for patiently guiding me through the tedious process of organizing the books and journal. But lastly, this book would not have been initiated if it was not for the idea and gentle nudge of my friend, Brian Hennessey. Brian is a student and also a published author who encouraged me to write this book. The final push came when he said, "You have something to say, so say it. It's already inside you. Get it out." This was exactly what I needed to hear to take the first steps into my next chapter.

About the Author

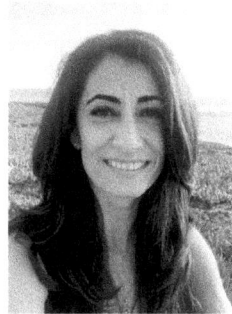

Mahnaz Jahangiri was born in December 1972 in Tehran, Iran. Her family came to The United States in the summer of 1977. Her parents soon decided on settling down in the small city of Westlake Village, north of Los Angeles.

She graduated from the California State University of Northridge and began her career in television game shows managing promotions and prizes for "Jeopardy!", "Wheel of Fortune" and "The Price is Right."

Mahnaz began her yoga practice in 1995 and in 1999 discovered Hot Yoga. After completing her first training in 2002, she began teaching in a small boutique studio in Encino, California. She soon found a strong desire to create her own space from the ground up. In 2007, she opened her first studio in a tree-lined office park in her hometown of Westlake Village. After her continued education in Vinyasa and Meditation courses, she started teacher trainings and, shortly after, opened a second studio in Korea Town, Los Angeles.

After over 10 years of operating the yoga studio(s), Mahnaz decided to shift the direction of her career again to teach privately to small groups and conduct workshops locally and in Lomas, Mexico City.

In March 2020, Mahnaz began teaching online classes and launched her first online membership site. The platform now offers over 500 classes including, yoga, meditation, mat Pilates and specialty classes. Mahnaz teaches live classes 7 days a week to students across the country.

To learn more, including information on memberships, visit www.samadiyoga.com.

www.ingramcontent.com/pod-product-compliance
Lightning Source LLC
Chambersburg PA
CBHW070117030426
42335CB00016B/2186

HEALING MUSHROOMS

A Comprehensive Guide to Using Medicinal Mushrooms

BARTON PRESS